CW01067482

Support for the bereaved and the dying

A guide for managers and staff in services for adults on the autism spectrum

Helen Green Allison

First published 2001 and reprinted 2014 by The National Autistic Society
393 City Road, London EC1V 1NG

www.autism.org.uk

The National Autistic Society is a charity registered in England and Wales (269425
and in Scotland (SC039427) and a company limited by guarantee registered in
England (No.1205298), registered office: 393 City Road, London EC1V 1NG.

ISBN 978 1 905722 82 2
Written by Helen Green Allison
Updated by Caroline Hattersley and Patrick Sims
Edited by Elizabeth Ayris
Designed by Cottier and Sidaway
Printed by Rap Spiderweb

Contents

Part 3: Supportive measures for
bereaved people with autism   41

Part 4: Other aspects of bereavement support   73

Part 5: Support for the dying   77

Preface

My paper, *The management of bereavement services for people with autism*, was written in 1992 with advice from managers of services for adults with autism. The introduction to that paper was as follows:

"Until recently, people with learning disabilities have been denied the right to grieve, on the mistaken assumption that they had no capacity to do so. This process of dehumanisation has been made all the more poignant by the movement towards advocating their rights in other areas (Kitching, 1987). Recognition both of their right and their capacity to grieve has led to a realisation that staff caring for people with learning disabilities should be trained to enable them, when they suffer loss, to complete the tasks of grieving in their own way and in their own time."

I hope that the right of people with autism not only to grieve but to be offered appropriate support in their grieving is now accepted in all services caring for them. However, I have revised my original work because of the impact of ageing on those cared for in services for adults: there is recognition of a greater need for preparation for bereavement management and the introduction of preparation for care of the dying. Increasing numbers of people with Asperger syndrome are now being diagnosed and terminology has also changed.

Much of the information regarding preparation for bereavement as well as strategies for support is still valid for the management of bereavement in children.

Appendix I, Grief reactions of people with autism, was compiled from the results of a survey undertaken as the basis for my original paper. It is no less valid at present than it was in 1992. Only one of those included was described as having Asperger syndrome, but it is likely that some of the others would now be similarly diagnosed.

Appendix II, Grief reactions of people with Asperger syndrome, was compiled from the results of a request for those who supported people with Asperger syndrome to supply information, similar to that in the first survey. Very few responses were received. However, I am grateful to those who did respond and to the young man with Asperger syndrome who offered a very moving analysis of his bereavement experience.

Helen Green Allison
2001

The purpose of this book

The main purpose of this book is to offer guidelines so that staff in services for people with autism can offer confident, informed and sensitive support to those they support in the event of bereavement.

There is a great deal of easily accessible literature on bereavement, and it is strongly recommended that staff familiarise themselves with the common responses to bereavement by referring to it (see Part 1, References and Useful contacts). This book will draw attention to the responses to bereavement of people with autism, and will suggest ways in which staff can train themselves in the management of bereavement, both in its practical aspects and in offering support to those who might be affected – including colleagues.

It cannot be overemphasised that because of the individual nature of reactions to bereavement and the grieving process, this book cannot be prescriptive. It can only suggest measures which can be adapted to individuals or from which a choice can be made.

Because support for the dying will become increasingly important in services for people with autism, it is hoped that some of the suggestions made in Part 5 may be helpful to staff who undertake this very demanding role.

Part 1: Bereavement management – the need for preparation

"There is no growth without pain and conflict and no loss that cannot lead to gain." (Pincus, 1961)

Introduction

The process of ageing is becoming ever more relevant to services caring for adults with autism. Therefore it follows that awareness of the issues surrounding bereavement – loss and death – is becoming an increasingly important component of the caring role as deaths of parents, of service staff and of people who use services themselves become more frequent. Accordingly, the need for staff to prepare themselves in order to offer effective practical and emotional support for people with autism through bereavement and death has become a matter of urgency.

The term 'autism' in this book is used to refer to:

"a lifelong developmental disability that affects how a person communicates with, and relates to, other people. It also affects how they make sense of the world around them.

"Autism is a spectrum condition, which means that, while all people with autism share certain difficulties, their condition will affect them in different ways. Some people with autism are able to live relatively independent lives but others may have accompanying learning disabilities and need a lifetime of specialist support. People with autism may also experience over- or under-sensitivity to sounds, touch, tastes, smells, light or colours.

"Asperger syndrome is a form of autism. People with Asperger syndrome are often of average or above average intelligence. They have fewer problems with speech but may still have difficulties with understanding and processing language."

For more information about autism, visit The National Autistic Society's website: www.autism.org.uk.

Throughout this book the term 'services' applies not only to residential and day establishments, but also to outreach services that support people with autism who live independently. In the interests of brevity, the term 'client' is used to describe a person who uses one or more of these services. The word 'parent' is used to refer to any person who fulfils a parental role in relation to a person who uses such services, including, for example, a significant family member or friend if there is no living or interested parent.

Responses to bereavement and grief

Bereavement and grief can be defined in many ways, but the experience will always be very individual. However it can be defined as 'a normal human emotion or set of emotions that occur in response to a significant loss' (Gulbenkoglu, 2007).

Studies of people with learning disabilities have shown that, of those who for no apparent reason suddenly presented with emotional and management difficulties, approximately half had experienced the death or loss of someone close before the change in behaviour (Emerson, 1977). Handley and Hutchinson (2012) found that in their study of people with 'intellectual disabilities' a change in behaviour could be noted in many after they had been told about the death of a family member. Similar results were shown in a study of admissions to an acute psychiatric ward of people with learning disabilities suffering from neurosis (Day, 1985). A limited cognitive capacity does not indicate a limited emotional capacity (Sireling, quoted in Kitchling, 1987). This view is also very much supported by Tuffrey-Wijne (2013).

We all respond differently to grief, whether or not we have a learning disability, but most of us share certain reactions. Because people with autism often find social interaction difficult, it might be thought that they do not form attachments to other people and are therefore insulated from the grieving process. It is true that statements have been made by individuals with autism (Schneider, 1999; Gillberg, 1991) which appear to confirm this. However, surveys undertaken of those who have supported people with autism through the grieving process have indicated that many have been deeply affected by the death of someone close (Appendix II and Rawlings, 1998). Marie Curie Cancer Care (2012) warns that the grief of someone with a learning disability can often be overlooked, misunderstood or ignored. The person may struggle, especially straightaway, to understand the news that a loved one has died. It is important to encourage them to ask questions about anything they don't understand (Marie Curie Cancer Care, 2012; Skylight Trust, 2007).

The examples available of people with autism who have successfully coped with grief are those who have received skilled support from family members or support staff. On the basis of these examples, five further conclusions can be reached.

1. All people with autism react individually to bereavement and the approach to support, if required, needs to be as unique as the individual involved.
2. A person may exhibit common responses to bereavement (see the next sub-section, The process of grieving) and may be affected by the major determinants of reactions to grief.
3. The grieving processes of people with autism are profoundly affected by their disabilities.
4. A person may undergo reactions similar to those of bereaved children and young people.
5. The problems and reactions of bereaved people with other learning disabilities may also be experienced by people with autism.

It follows that training resources and publications relating to bereavement in children and people with learning disabilities may be helpful to those supporting people with autism.

The process of grieving

Any or all of the following responses to grief may be experienced by bereaved people. Many experts, such as Kübler-Ross (2005), view grief as a process with identifiable stages which may include:

- shock, numbness, denial
- despair, turmoil and acute grieving, including:
    - anger
    - guilt

- anxiety, fear, panic
- depression
- pain, appetite disturbance, breathlessness, illness
- more than usual need for sleep, sleeplessness, hyperactivity
- nightmares
- regression, loss of skills
- recovery
- acceptance
- resolution of grief
- when the bereaved can think of the deceased without pain or anger and can recall the times they had together in a positive way.

These concepts are helpful, provided it is understood that people do not experience an orderly progression from one stage to the other. The stages are, instead, responses which may overlap and merge with each other (Carr, 1988). The shock/denial stage may last for hours or weeks. The other stages last longer and have no time limit. Normally, mourning the loss of a close relationship takes a year and may take as long as two years (Worden, 1991).

Acceptance and recovery do not imply that grief is over. It can be felt throughout life, sometimes as a stab of pain, but also in the form of a memory of shared experience. Anniversaries are particularly difficult – for example, the date of the death, birthdays, festivals such as Christmas and other celebrations which might have been shared with the deceased.

In her book for professionals, *Loss and learning disability* (2003), Noelle Blackman discusses how to prevent 'normal' grief from becoming a larger problem and how to support people when the process 'goes wrong'.

The intensity and duration of a person's responses to grief are affected by a combination of important factors. Who the deceased was and the closeness of the relationship to the bereaved is of great importance. The nature of the attachment, its strength and security, or the ambivalence of the relationship, including any conflicts during the lifetime of the deceased, may influence a person's reaction.

The mode of death – whether it occurred suddenly or with advance warning – has an impact, too. It is usually easier to accept the death of a person ripe in years than that of a young person. Natural deaths are more easily accepted than accidental deaths; suicides and homicides are particularly hard to accept (Wertheimer, 2001). Another factor is where the death happened geographically, whether nearby or far away.

Historical factors also play a part. A bereaved person's previous experiences of grieving – for example, the irresolution of a previous death – may affect reactions to a subsequent death. Those with a history of depression may have increased difficulty in coping with bereavement. This is an extremely important point to be aware of as there is a much higher prevalence of depression in people with autism than in the rest of the population – approximately 30% (Madders, 2010; Sims, 2011).

The personality, age and sex of a bereaved individual will also influence their response. So, too, will their ability to handle anxiety and stress, whether they have difficulty in expressing themselves, whether they are highly dependent, or if they have problems forming relationships. People diagnosed with certain personality disorders may find it difficult to cope with loss.

Social variables are significant, too. Cultural and religious backgrounds, including grieving rituals, as well as the degree of perceived emotional and social support from others, influence the responses of the bereaved. Their lives may be further affected during the grieving process by other stressful, disruptive and possibly life-changing events following the death.

Relating responses to grief to those with autism

Staff wishing to offer support to a bereaved individual need to bear in mind the major factors that may determine responses to grief. They also need to be aware of the ways that a person's autism may affect their grieving process. These factors will be discussed in various contexts in this book, but it should be pointed out here that, because autism affects people in different ways and to different degrees, this introduces an additional complexity into the functions of staff offering support to bereaved clients. For example, a more able individual may require detailed explanations and the opportunity to explore their own concepts of death and after-life beliefs. Those in the mid-range would probably derive most comfort from simple, factual, directive language. Those who are very severely affected, perhaps with accompanying learning difficulties, might be confused by anything but the minimum information. Staff must be prepared, therefore, to respond flexibly, depending on the individual who is bereaved (Tuffrey-Wijne, 2013).

Specific grief reactions of people with autism are described in the appendices. It is important to bear these in mind as they may help staff to interpret the reactions of those they support.

Types of bereavement

Bereavement in services for people with autism may take a variety of forms – not simply relating to the death of a loved one.

Bereavement may also happen if a person has to move home (perhaps because their parents' marriage breaks up), or if siblings move away from the family home. A transfer from one living environment to another and staff changes, or the loss of a pet or of a precious possession may have a profound impact, too.

The greater part of this book is concerned with the loss of a family member. The loss of a second parent can be particularly difficult to accept because of the fundamental life changes which may follow. The death of another person who uses the service or a staff member may also affect a person with autism – perhaps profoundly. Most of the suggestions in this book can therefore apply in this context as well.

Ageing parents: ways to maintain family contact

Before giving details of the preparations for bereavement management itself, it is important to outline the problems faced by ageing parents and the ways in which services can help both client and parent maintain their relationship.

Safeguards for the lone parent

As people with autism age it becomes more likely, either because of death or divorce, that they will be left with just one parent who will be their sole carer during home visits. This poses the risk that, should the parent become seriously ill or incapacitated, the person with autism will be left alone, lacking the ability to call for help.

Accordingly, staff in services should make sure that someone suitable is found to support the parent when their child visits them at home. Should this not be possible, suggest that the parent makes an agreement with a staff member or a reliable friend or relative to telephone them at an agreed time every day. Alternatively, the parent could telephone someone every day at an agreed time. If contact is not made, staff, relatives or friends can immediately take whatever action is necessary.

Supporting parents in a changing situation

As parents age they will inevitably have diminished stamina and perhaps age-related disabilities. They may start to find it difficult or impossible to drive or to travel on public transport to visit their child. Or, they may not feel able to manage the home visits that have been an important part of their lives and their child's. Ending home visits at Christmas, Easter and birthdays can be traumatic for both parties.

This problem should not be allowed to erode family relationships. While a meaningful telephone conversation with a person with autism may not be an option, new technology could offer alternative means of communication which should be encouraged where appropriate.

Staff can take an active role in preserving family relationships by providing support during home visits, taking families on outings together, or making arrangements for parents to visit the service. You might book local overnight accommodation for parents who live some distance away. Alternatively, services, where possible, can provide guest accommodation for parents on the premises.

Part 2: Preparation for bereavement management

Preparation is key

When preparing your approach to bereavement management, try to have some clear objectives in mind. Essential components of the planning process include putting a sound set of procedures in place, working with an individual's family where possible and sensitive staff training.

Strategies to support an individual and involve their family include the following.

- Make sure that relevant information about all the people you support is available in the event of bereavement or death. This should include details of previous losses, people's cultural and religious backgrounds, contact details of significant persons and forms of address used by people for those close to them (for example 'Mum' rather than 'Mother').
- Encourage parents to plan the rituals surrounding their own deaths so that they are meaningful for their son or daughter. Tell staff about measures which will help to provide comfort when bereavement occurs.
- Encourage parents to plan for the welfare of their son or daughter after their deaths, in particular by financial planning and provision of supportive relationships. Facilitate other supportive relationships.
- Be prepared to offer help to other family members in understanding, or at least coming to terms with, the reactions to bereavement of people you support.

- Make sure that bereaved clients are supported by designated members of staff who know them well and who understand the grieving process.
- Invite parents to record their wishes in respect of the death of their son or daughter and, if possible, make sure that funds are available for a funeral and burial, or cremation arrangements.
- Be prepared to undertake the necessary practical arrangements following the death of a person you support.
- Be prepared to offer support to family members if a person you support dies.

Training measures for service staff to help their bereaved clients include the following.

- Knowledge of bereavement management in this context: this means a sound understanding of autism and of the people you support, their personalities and significant facts about them; knowing how to make appropriate funeral arrangements; and understanding how to approach and support relatives.
- The ability to explain or talk about loss and death with the people you support, if and when they are bereaved, and help them to cope.
- The ability to offer practical help to people who have been bereaved, for example making the rituals of death more meaningful to an individual, supporting them in their own way of grieving, and in forming concepts of death and after-life beliefs.

It is also important to support staff while they are caring for a person who is facing death – and when coping with their own potential grief after the person dies. Marie Curie Cancer Care produces a document called *Bereavement: helping you deal with the death on someone close to you*. It is free to download from www. mariecurie.org.uk/resources and would make excellent reference material for all service managers.

While aiming to meet these objectives, there is an understanding that all bereavements are unique and that staff will decide which strategies are appropriate in different circumstances.

Forming a bereavement support group

Bereavement support groups in services are one of the recommended ways of introducing successful bereavement management, monitoring it and making sure that standards of bereavement training are met.

Members of a bereavement support group could include staff who have received bereavement training, local clergy and other religious figures, professionals from organisations such as Cruse Bereavement Care, The Compassionate Friends or the Samaritans, and relatives.

Bereavement questionnaires

Collecting relevant information about the people you support, and encouraging parents to make arrangements for their son or daughter after their death, can help considerably with managing bereavement.

A bereavement questionnaire should include the following sections.

1. Factual information which will help staff to offer effective support, including previous losses that a person has experienced, how parents want their son or daughter to be told about their deaths, where to get advice so that the person can take part in the rituals surrounding death, and the forms of address the person uses for those close to them.
2. Financial provision for people who use services, whether through a will or settlement, and how it can be accessed on their behalf by the service.
3. The names and contact details of people who have been nominated to perform some roles previously provided by parents, such as home visits, friendship and advocacy.
4. Parents' wishes in respect of arrangements following the death of their family member.
5. Family members' views on death (if these have been expressed).

A sample questionnaire, which can be adapted for use for adults, is available from www.autism.org.uk/bereavementquestionnaire.

Although it is desirable that the questionnaire be completed by parents when their son or daughter joins a service, it can be done in stages as families' plans for the future develop. Completed questionnaires should be kept in confidential files and periodically reviewed, possibly at regular review meetings, so that they can be updated as necessary.

Encouraging parents to consider their own funeral arrangements

Encourage parents to consider their own funeral arrangements, so that they are meaningful to their son or daughter and they are able to participate. Staff can talk with parents about how this might be achieved, perhaps when parents are completing a bereavement questionnaire.

Staff may need to remind parents, particularly those who want their remains to be cremated, that some people with autism might benefit from a focus for their grieving process. For example, a memorial stone which they can visit and where they can plant a rose bush or lay flowers.

Encouraging parents to make provision for the welfare of their son or daughter

It is extremely important that staff communicate effectively and regularly with parents about financial issues. It is wise for parents to prepare for the welfare of their son or daughter after their own deaths: this might include looking at settlements, wills and trusts. Financial and legal advice changes, so we recommend visiting the following websites for up-to-date information:

- www.autism.org.uk/will
- www.mariecurie.org.uk
- www.mencap.org.uk/what-we-do/wills-and-trusts (Mencap also has a wills and trusts advice service which offers free access to a solicitor).

Financial arrangements should be recorded appropriately (check current best practice) so that there is a permanent record accessible to staff at the time of parents' deaths.

Supportive relationships

In the event of the death or incapacity of parents, supportive relationships can be established with other people. They can take the form either of a 'successor parent' who takes over parents' caring and advocacy roles, or a 'citizen advocate' who, strictly speaking, serves as an advocate for an individual but may also serve in a caring role. To be effective, both functions must be undertaken by people considerably closer in age to an individual than their parents. It is helpful if supportive relationships are established while parents can brief people about their role and familiarise them with the aims of the service that cares for their son or daughter.

Successor parent

A successor parent is usually a person's sibling, a relative or a family friend. They should have expressed a clear wish to serve in this capacity. Whether or not siblings have been chosen as successor parents, staff will wish to build up a relationship between siblings and their brother or sister. This should be done sensitively as some siblings may not wish to be involved. The term 'successor parent' is used in preference to 'befriender' because the former implies a long-term commitment to undertake aspects of the parental role. This in no way denigrates befrienders, who can help to enrich the life of a person with autism by providing companionship.

Advocacy

The *Mental Capacity Act 2005*, which applies to England and Wales, makes it a legal requirement to ensure all people with a learning disability, mental health difficulty and dementia have their views and wishes heard. In Scotland, the *Adults with Incapacity (Scotland) Act 2000* provides a legal basis for safeguarding adults (age 16 and over) who lack capacity to act or make some or all decisions for themselves. If a person is deemed not to have capacity, they have the right to non-instructed advocacy so that decisions and actions can be made on their behalf, if seen to be in their best interest. A specially trained advocate will get to know an individual and attempt to find out if they have a particular wish, need or requirement (Department of Health 2005a; Medley and Saunders, 2006). The advocate must be independent and focused on the needs of the person they are working with or for (Parsons and Sims, 2010).

Staff, with the consent of parents, may need to take part in selecting and appointing citizen advocates. As soon as a citizen advocate is appointed, they will have a standing in relation to a person with autism which must be recognised. A conscientious citizen advocate will wish to get to know an individual well so that he or she can represent them effectively.

Building a supportive relationship

While a person's parents are alive staff should, in cooperation with them, take measures to build supportive relationships. The goal is a seamless transfer of caring and advocacy roles if parents die or become incapacitated.

Staff can welcome visits by a successor parent or citizen advocate and let them know that they are free to discuss (in private) the client's personality and interests, whether by telephone or during visits to the service. Keep successor parents and advocates informed of an individual's activities, and invite them to annual review meetings, parent partnership meetings and any other meetings where you discuss an individual's progress and future development. You can also include their names on mailing lists for your newsletter, if you have one, and any important notices.

Parents' wishes in respect of the death of their son or daughter

Bereavement questionnaires (see page 21) invite parents to record their wishes in respect of the death of their son or daughter. It is clearly beneficial if parents make sure that funds are available for a funeral and burial or cremation.

Parents may prefer to make these funds available through a pre-paid funeral plan or by a will or settlement. Undertaking firms can give advice about pre-paid plans. The service must do its best to fulfil parents' stated wishes concerning the type of funeral service (religious, secular or humanist), burial or cremation arrangements and preferred type of memorial.

If parents are still living when their son or daughter dies and they, or other relatives, want to be involved in funeral arrangements, it is hoped that they will reach an agreement with staff on how the responsibility will be shared.

Practical arrangements following the death of a person you support

Services that support adults with autism must be prepared to take responsibility for practical arrangements if and when a person dies. This includes notification and registration of death, as well as facilitating the funeral and burial or cremation.

If a death is reported to the coroner, there may be a post mortem examination of the body and possibly an inquest. Marie Curie Cancer Care's booklet, *Bereavement: helping you to deal with the death of someone close to you*, is free to download and a really practical guide. See www.mariecurie.org.uk.

Religious and ethnic background of the deceased

When a person dies and before any action is taken regarding the laying out of the body and the rituals surrounding death, close regard must be paid to their religious and ethnic background. Different religions have their own practices regarding the preparation of the body and its burial or cremation. If you do not already have links with local religious organisations or figures it is important to contact someone, so that the rituals surrounding a person's death are appropriate.

Taking primary responsibility for funeral arrangements

If a service has to take primary responsibility for the funeral arrangements of a person it has supported, it may be wise for staff to get in touch with several local undertakers. They can then find out what is involved and which options are available. Staff should be aware that undertaking is a business and that efforts may be made to sell as many services as possible.

When arranging a funeral, obtain at least two estimates and compare costs. There can be a great deal of flexibility in funeral arrangements, and it is possible to organise a simple, dignified and relatively inexpensive funeral in which mourners can take an active part.

Cruse Bereavement Care (2013) says that a good training strategy is for staff to visit an undertaker (making it clear that it is part of a training exercise) to negotiate the type of funeral that they, personally, would like to have. It would be positive if staff ask someone who is not directly involved in funeral planning to accompany them, to give an objective view and to support them in requesting time to think about the options before making a decision. Staff may also find it helpful to attend an open day at a crematorium so that they know what to expect if they have to arrange a cremation.

Getting to know the local vicar, priest or religious leader

A local vicar, priest or religious leader can be a valuable source of advice when making arrangements for a funeral, burial, cremation or memorial service. They may also be able to help support bereaved individuals or staff. You may already have established links with religious leaders by regular attendance at services and, if willing, a religious representative can become a valuable member of a bereavement support group, and perhaps help with staff training on bereavement management.

Preparing staff to manage bereavement

It is essential that staff supporting people with autism through the grieving process should not only understand common responses to bereavement, but also autism, the personalities of individuals they support, any previous losses people have experienced, and any close or important relationships they have. This will help staff to interpret the reactions of a bereaved person, and also to provide support in ways which can circumvent the barriers of their disabilities. This knowledge will help make staff training in bereavement more effective.

Knowledge of autism and communication strategies

Services should give staff access to suitable training courses and make literature on autism available in various formats, so that they are aware how autism may affect the grieving process. There is, however, no substitute for hands-on experience.

Through training, staff should be able to increase their understanding of the use of non-verbal communication with people with autism. This includes the use of signs, symbols and photographs – all of which can be usefully combined with each other as well as with verbal communication (Parsons and Sims, 2010). These approaches can be used by staff when offering bereavement support. Staff trained in the use of social stories™ or comic strip conversations (Gray, 1998; Gray Center, 2013) which are descriptive and visual methods for teaching people with autism about social situations, may find these useful when supporting bereaved individuals. Tuffrey-Wijne (2013) also recommends drawing pictures as a way of starting a conversation and of allowing people to describe how they are feeling.

Understanding individual clients

Personalities

It is impossible to offer effective support to a bereaved person with autism without understanding their individual personality. This knowledge can be acquired only over a period of time by supporting them and observing them carefully, by communicating with parents and by consulting professionals who previously cared for them. Staff should familiarise themselves with the person's life story and past experiences.

Previous losses: impact on subsequent bereavements

When a person is bereaved, the pain of an earlier loss may be reactivated or actually be felt for the first time, because it may never have been resolved (Worden, 1991). It is therefore important for staff to learn as much as possible about a person's previous losses and bereavements; when they happened, how they were managed and how the individual reacted. Consultation with parents and professionals who have supported them in the past can be helpful.

The types of losses likely to have been experienced by adults with autism are given in Part 1. They may include losses other than the death of someone close, such as those resulting from transition and staff changes.

Significant facts

It is important to have easily accessible, and specific personal information on file about the people you support, not only for general purposes but also for use if they are bereaved. This information should include:

- the cultural and religious beliefs and traditions of the individual and their family
- contact details of family members and other important people, such as family friends, a citizen advocate or a befriender
- contact details of social workers, doctors and any other professionals involved with a person.

These facts can be helpful when staff need to take practical measures following the death of a person they support, a member of a person's family or a close friend. Bereavement questionnaires can be a good way to assemble these details.

Forms of address

To help manage bereavement effectively, staff should have access not only to the names, addresses and relationships of family members, but also a note of how they are addressed by the person with autism. It is no good consoling an individual for the death of 'Dad' if he was known as 'Father', 'Nan' if she was known as 'Granny', 'Mum' if she was known as 'Mummy' or 'Catherine' if she was known as 'Kate'.

Religious and cultural backgrounds

An understanding of people's religious and cultural traditions is essential for staff involved in the management of bereavement: it will help them confidently and sensitively to support an individual in the grieving process by drawing on concepts acceptable to the family and from the person's own upbringing. Staff can prepare the individual for what to expect and, where necessary, accompany to the funeral and other ceremonies.

When a person dies who has been using a service, staff may be involved in making arrangements for a funeral or a memorial service. Staff may therefore need to seek information on religious and cultural customs and rituals from family members and local religious leaders. They are likely to discover that such people are pleased to be of help.

Religion and cultural topics are included in *Understanding grief* by Sheila Hollins and Lester Sireling (1999) an in-house training course for those caring for people with learning disabilities who have been bereaved. A useful book covering rites, rituals and mourning traditions for the major religious and secular belief systems is *Death and bereavement across cultures* (edited by Colin Murray Parkes, Pittu Laugani and Bill Young, 1997).

Information on humanist and non-religious funerals and cremations can be obtained from the British Humanist Association or the National Secular Society (see the section Useful contacts).

Training staff to provide loss and death education

There are comparatively few resources on educating people about loss and death, so that they manage their own feelings in the event of future bereavements. Resources include the following:

- www.breakingbadnews.org a website designed to support professionals in breaking bad news to people with 'intellectual disabilities' that they are working with (checked March 2013)
- Tuffrey-Winje, I. (2013). *How to break bad news to people with intellectual disabilities.* London: Jessica Kingsley Publishers.
- Hollins, S. and Tuffrey-Wijne, I. (2009). *Am I going to die?* London: RSPsych Publications/St George's, University of London.

Preparing people with autism for loss and bereavement

Education about loss and death for children and people with learning disabilities, when developmentally appropriate, helps to make it less difficult for them to deal with bereavement when the time comes (Ward et al, 1996; Hollins and Sireling, 1999). The same applies to people with autism. It must be undertaken with caution and an understanding of the individual concerned.

Because of the individuality of people with autism, their varying levels of cognition and emotional maturity, and often high levels of anxiety, it is likely that preparation will need to happen informally, on an individual basis and when appropriate opportunities present themselves.

Saying goodbye: endings and new beginnings

People with autism will experience a number of losses in everyday life and, if they have been prepared to handle these 'little deaths', may become more able to cope with major bereavements.

People with autism will need to be made aware of saying goodbye to things and people in their lives, and encouraged to respond positively to new situations. For example, some people find it difficult to leave their families at the end of home visits. Help them to overcome their distress by encouraging them to look forward to pleasurable activities back at their service, as well as future home visits.

Another common loss that people with autism in services experience is the departure of staff. This can provide opportunities to experience the rituals of farewell, such as parties and gifts. It can be argued that because of the effects on those they support, staff should be careful not to let ties become too strong – but if the ties are those of friendship with no pathological overtones, discouraging them will deprive individuals of real-life experiences. A person with autism could, potentially, keep in contact with staff who have left by telephone calls, letters and visits. Point out that these actions can help to convert loss into gain.

Memory books

Memory books, or life story books, are visual records of experiences which have been important to people. If a person you support is capable of doing so and it is appropriate, you could encourage them to make one. Parents and other significant people should be invited to contribute.

The book could include pictures of happy incidents in a person's life, family holidays, previous homes, letters and postcards from loved ones and photographs of family members and pets. Film of family activities might be helpful, too, but should be used with caution. It may cause confusion about the finality of death.

As well as giving pleasure, these books - with assistance from staff - may help a person to understand the concepts of the flow of life and of ageing. They may also help with the grieving process in due course, and with reminiscing about family members or pets who have died.

Explaining death to people with autism

Opportunities should be taken to explain death simply and factually, as part of the life cycle, without speculation or prediction. There are some very good examples of supporting people with learning disabilities to understand and plan for their deaths. In his book, *When I die*, Tony Johnston clearly sets out his wishes for his deteriorating health, death and funeral (see www. easyhealth.org.uk).

It is important not to present death to a person with communication difficulties or learning disabilities as it happens. Instead, work up to it over a period of time using examples such as plants, insects or pets dying (Tuffrey-Wijne, 2013). You could also talk about the deaths of people who are not close to a person, such as public figures or acquaintances. There may be circumstances when it is appropriate for a person to write letters of condolence or to send flowers to bereaved people who are in their circle of friends or wider acquaintance. For example, people who go to special schools may experience the deaths of class mates (Tuffrey-Wijne, 2013). The same author suggests that some people will not be able to understand the notion of death and bereavement until they experience it so it is imperative that support staff, carers and others work together to support them.

It is likely that many people with autism will have difficulty in grasping the components of the concept of death:

- inevitability – the realisation that life comes to an end
- irreversibility – the permanence of death
- non-functionality – the body ceasing to function
- universality – the fact that it happens to all living creatures (Cathcart, 1994; Kane, 1997; Read et al, 2012).

All of the major world religions believe in the continuation of the soul after death. Hindus, Buddhists and Sikhs believe in reincarnation (that the soul returns as a new person many times). Christians, Jews and Muslims believe that a person lives only once and that after death their soul will go to heaven or hell.

Personally, you may be uncertain whether death is the final end or whether there is such a thing as immortality. If a person you support is concerned about this, the book *Good grief (2)* (1998) advises that it is better to say, 'No one yet knows, but people are still trying to find out' than to say, 'I don't know'. Staff with strong religious beliefs or strong atheist convictions must recognise that these are their personal views and not let them affect the way they support the bereaved.

Good grief (2) includes a section in which beliefs about death are simply explained. This can be summarised as follows and may be adapted for people with autism.

There are two aspects of death: the body and the spiritual aspect.

What happens to the body can be understood by children if it is explained simply – that the dead person cannot have feelings, cannot feel hot or cold, hurt or sick. Their dead body is of no use to them. A simple explanation is then given of cremation and burial (Skylight Trust, 2007).

With the spiritual aspect, the following ideas are considered.

- There is no continuance of the individual spirit.
- There is a continuation in some form. People die when they have done the work they have to do, but life may continue in a different way. Some children have found the concept of the life cycle of insects helpful (see *Waterbugs and dragonflies* by Doris Stickney, 1984) or even the concept of the persistence of atoms and electrons after the cremation of the body.
- There are differing points of view on the religious aspects of the soul and spirit. Abstract religious ideas are not necessarily helpful and Christian concepts are particularly difficult to understand. Children find it easier to come to terms with pantheism and reincarnation.

The chapter goes on to discuss three aspects of death of particular concern to children, which can be adapted for people with autism as appropriate.

- Are dead people sleeping? A clear distinction should be made between sleep and death. Sleep gives rest and renewal. Death is when the body stops working.
- What happens to dead people? Our bodies wear out. Our spirit or soul, which enables us to give and receive love, never wears out. We cannot see it, but people of all religions (and in some cases those of no religion) believe it lives on after we die. The analogy is offered of a person leaving a house, which then ceases to be a home.
- What is heaven like? The spirit or soul no longer experiences the sadness and troubles we have on Earth. It goes to heaven which is where God is. Because God is love, heaven is a place full of love. No-one knows what heaven looks like or where it is (Hayworth, 1996).

It may be that these concepts are too difficult for some people with autism to understand. The most effective explanations of death are those which are simple and which draw as far as possible on an individual's own experiences. Their level of understanding must dictate the pace. When discussing concepts of death, staff must be careful not to confuse those they support with ideas that might conflict with their cultural backgrounds. Bear in mind too that introducing a discussion which may cause anxiety in a person with autism can be counter-productive.

Anxiety and misconceptions about death

People with autism may become fearful and anxious about death. This anxiety may arise in different ways. A person may be unconcerned about the death of older people such as grandparents, but anxious when they hear of deaths in their own age group. If they have lost one member of their immediate family, especially a parent, they may be fearful of losing remaining family members. They may feel threatened by deaths represented on television.

You may need to reassure those you support, playing down the likelihood of their imminent death or the death of family members or, if appropriate, drawing on the concepts of the continuation of life in some form. There is a particular need for staff to be vigilant in regard to high-functioning people with autism, and especially those with Asperger syndrome, who may become obsessed with the idea of death and even of taking their own lives.

People with autism can, sometimes, have bizarre and distorted ideas of death. For example, a young school leaver was convinced that his own death was imminent. He knew that a member of staff had died and had 'left the premises'; he had also watched older pupils depart, never to be seen again. When staff discovered the source of his anxiety, they were able to arrange for him to speak to those pupils who had left, who told him about their life in a new setting.

Staff should try to identify any misunderstanding about death and work out its source and nature by sensitive questioning and observation, in order to tackle it effectively.

Training staff to support clients when bereavement occurs

Effective support for bereaved individuals relies in the first instance on staff understanding the common responses to bereavement and causes of grief. They can then relate these to the grieving processes of the people they support, and understand how autism may affect the process.

There is a wide variety of training resources available. See the References section for full details of the books and resources mentioned in this chapter.

Part 3: Supportive measures for bereaved people with autism

Designating members of staff to support bereaved clients

If a person you support is grieving, make sure they are supported by designated members of staff who understand the grieving process and have a good relationship with the person. They should also know the person's usual behaviour and be able to observe differences (Handley and Hutchinson, 2012).

When deciding who should undertake this role, consult those who know the person best, including family members if possible. If a death is anticipated, use the extra time you have to select suitable staff and to remind them of the issues that may be involved. The most important factors when selecting staff are looking at the relationship they have with the person with autism, and their ability to feel comfortable when talking about death.

Ideally a key worker, assisted by another staff member who knows the individual well, would serve in this capacity. However, there may be good reasons why staff do not wish to undertake this role, such as a lack of experience of bereavement, or concern that a bereavement of their own might be brought to the surface again. No-one who has suffered a recent bereavement should be called upon to support a bereaved client.

Bereavement support workers need not necessarily be a member of support staff. They could be maintenance or office staff if a person has a particular affinity with them.

Bereavement support workers should be prepared to:

- keep all staff who come into contact with the person informed of their reactions to bereavement and of any special needs they may have at that time
- help a person participate in the rituals surrounding death, preferably with the agreement of their family
- provide comfort and facilitate the grieving process.

Because of staff rotas, it is not possible for a support worker, or even the person who assists them, to be on duty at all times during the bereavement process, which may last more than two years. All staff who play a part in supporting a person should have access at all times to someone, preferably a member of the bereavement support group, who can give them guidance.

Anticipated or sudden death: informing the client

Anticipated death

Although it is not conclusive, there is some evidence that if death is anticipated, the grieving process is less difficult for the bereaved than in the case of sudden death (Parkes, 1996). However, anticipated death can lead to pre-death bereavement and can also be a source of acute anxiety (Worden, 1991). Staff will therefore wish to consider carefully, in the light of their knowledge of an individual, whether or not they should be informed of an impending death. If at all possible, discuss the matter with family members before making a decision. One young man with autism who knew that his father had a weak heart was able to accept his death when he was told that his father had died of a heart attack, although he suffered acute grief reactions.

Visiting the dying

Giving a person you support the opportunity to visit their dying relative in hospital and say goodbye may help them to accept the finality of death. It can also help the grieving process (see *When Dad died* by Hollins and Sireling, 1999, in which a son visits his dying father). Talk to family members about whether it is in a person's best interests to visit, bearing in mind that some might find the occasion unduly stressful or an additional source of anxiety. It may be unwise to plan a visit if the patient is on a drip or receiving visible life support.

If you are going ahead with a hospital visit, prepare carefully. Make sure that any staff members escorting a person with autism are confident about carrying out the difficult task of visiting someone who is terminally ill. Brief the person with autism themselves so that they know what to expect, possibly discussing any changes such as the dying person becoming weaker or unable to communicate (Booklet 3, Cathcart, 1994).

The visit need not be a long one and conversation is not necessary: a person with autism could simply sit beside the patient, perhaps taking his or her hand. It may be appropriate to encourage an individual to give the dying person a present, as long as they realise that this will not help them to recover (Booklet 3, Cathcart, 1994).

Sudden death

Sudden death can devastate a service. Those affected suffer profound shock; they experience the natural stages of grief but in a more acute and amplified form.

Small services are particularly vulnerable and need access to an independent support network of people who are not grieving themselves. Both staff and people who use the service may find it difficult to re-enter the home, particularly the room of the deceased. Some staff may have anxieties about undertaking sleeping-in duties and some residents may need to take comfort in room-sharing for a time, where appropriate and safe.

It is vitally important that news of the death is communicated speedily to everyone who is likely to be affected by it – for example, other people who use the service, staff, parents and professionals – and that they do not learn about it from chatter and hearsay. The service should be prepared to offer support and reassurance to all those affected by the death. (For advice on how to break the news, see the section Who should tell clients about a death?)

A sudden death is likely to lead to a post-mortem and inquest. If this is the case, there will be a delay before funeral arrangements can be finalised. This will be a period of disquiet for everyone affected, especially those who were providing hands-on support.

In the main, this section refers to the death of a person with autism who uses a service, but the principles could also apply to the sudden death of a staff member or parent.

Initiating bereavement management

Who should tell clients about a death?

This decision should be thought through carefully. Should people be told by someone in their family, or by a staff member? (if a family member or someone close to the family has died, the decision should be reached in consultation with the family.) Parents are occasionally unwilling to tell their son or daughter about a death, in order to avoid the devastating impact on them but, however well-intentioned, withholding information cannot be considered good practice.

It is possible that the person who breaks bad news may become the target of aggression, if a bereaved person is angry. It may not be wise, for example, to let a mother undertake this task if she lives on her own with her child. For the same reason, if a member of staff breaks bad news, it might not be appropriate for them to support the bereaved while they grieve. When breaking the news in a service, choose a quiet location where there will be no interruptions. The informant should also be supported by another staff member.

How to inform a client

Staudacher (1988) gives some practical advice on how to inform a child about death. This advice is adapted here for people with autism.

- Use forms of communication appropriate to a person's level of understanding. Tell the truth, without giving unnecessary or disturbing details.

- Do not expect a person to respond in an 'acceptable' way (for example, with overt sadness).
- Observe how a person appears to be feeling.
- Allow them to release their feelings.
- Allow them to take the lead and ask questions (in some circumstances they may need sensitive prompting).
- Answer all questions readily and honestly. If there is no answer, say 'No one knows' and if an answer is not immediately available, try to obtain it as soon as possible.
- Reassure them that their daily routine will go on and that they will continue to be supported (if this is the case and bearing in mind that home visits may have to cease).
- Show affection and support.

Terms in which death should be explained

A simple, factual description of death is recommended for both children and those with learning disabilities (Schaeffer and Lyons, 1998; Hollins and Sireling, 1999; Skylight Trust, 2007) along the lines of: His/her body won't work any more. It can't move, talk, walk, see or hear. He/she is not asleep, has stopped breathing, can't eat, drink, feel hot or cold.

There should be no suggestion that there is hope of return (though in some circumstances mention may be made of reincarnation) and euphemisms such as 'gone to sleep', 'left us,' and 'you have lost your father/mother' should be avoided as they may lead to confusion and distress. In some cases, it may be helpful to ask an individual to repeat what they have been told.

If a person has any misapprehensions about the nature or causes of death, these should be cleared up immediately. For example, after his father's death, one school-age boy developed an obsession for rushing upstairs wherever he was, in order to get to the attic or roof space. It transpired that his brother, when talking about his father's death, had pointed upwards and said that he was 'up there'. The boy had interpreted this to mean that his father was in the attic (Jordan and Powell, 1995).

The tendency of people with autism to interpret things literally must always be taken into account. Avoid saying that a dead person has 'gone to a better place' and make it clear that living is desirable. A doctrinaire stance is necessary in this instance to prevent preoccupation with suicide (Rawlings, 1998).

The ability of an individual to understand accurately what they are told about death may affect the way they work through the normal grieving process (McLoughlin, 1986). Staff can help by doing everything in their power to give those they support an understanding of the death at a level at which it can be absorbed. Viewing the body can be the most effective means of accomplishing this. One young woman, who was taken to view her mother's body after death, appeared to understand immediately the irreversibility of death. Having been unable to wake her mother, she sighed, 'empty, all gone'. Meanwhile, a profoundly disabled young woman without speech was helped to learn about her mother's death by being shown a photograph of her previously deceased father and given her mother's clothes to handle (Oswin, 1991). For non-verbal individuals the use of signs, symbols and photographs can be useful in explaining death. For example, a service which kept a correspondence file with photographs of family and friends helped one person to accept the death of his grandmother by transferring her photographs from the file into a special album.

Discuss the terms you use to explain death with a person's family, and make every effort to comply with their wishes. Families' advice may, in fact, run counter to the recommendation of a purely factual explanation of death, but if a family wants an individual to be told the deceased 'has gone to heaven' or 'is with Jesus', their wish should be respected. You can point out that confusion may arise if the person you support views the body or attends the funeral, cremation or burial. There are examples, however, of successful resolution of grief by people with autism who have been told that the deceased has gone to heaven, and subsequently participated in the bereavement rituals. Some individuals have seemed to accept 'gone to heaven' as a factual explanation of someone having gone to a specific place where they themselves cannot at present go. Others have found comfort in the concept of reincarnation. There is no doubt that a number of people with autism have derived benefit from after-life beliefs (see Appendix).

If a person you support has experienced a previous bereavement, it is important to explain any subsequent death in the same terms. Again, the family may need to be consulted.

Explaining the cause of death

The four categories of death – natural, accidental, suicidal and homicidal – and the type of death can all have an effect on the grieving process (Worden, 1991). The first two types of death are more easily explained to a person with autism. People with autism sometimes ask where or when someone died, but seldom ask how, although staff should be prepared for them to do so. Those who do ask 'how' may be better able to assimilate the answer.

In explaining death, it is important always to be honest and consistent, without giving details which are unnecessary or disturbing (Staudacher, 1988). Natural deaths can be explained by saying that the deceased was very old so his/her body wore out and stopped working (Schaeffer and Lyons,1998; Skylight Trust, 2007) or that they were fatally (or terminally) ill and the doctor could not make them better. Care should be taken when mentioning illness to avoid using the expression 'very ill', as this might later be used when an individual themselves is ill. They may then believe that they are on the point of death.

An accidental death can be explained by saying that a person's body was so badly hurt that the doctor could not make it better, so it stopped working (Schaeffer and Lyons, 1998).

Bereavement advice relating to children who are being told of a death by suicide emphasises that they should be told the truth simply and honestly. Experience has shown that they are likely to find out indirectly or to realise that they are not being told the truth, with severe adverse consequences in either case. If there is no doubt that the deceased planned to kill themselves, the death should be explained to a child along the following lines: 'Sometimes a person's mind doesn't work right. They can't see things clearly and they felt the only way to solve their problems was by ending their life' (Schaeffer and Lyons, 1998). This might not be an appropriate explanation to offer to a person with autism. A more able person is likely to ask how the death occurred and might even ask if it was done on purpose. On the other hand, there are dangers in telling them about a suicide because there is a high level of severe depression in this group, sometimes leading to suicide. It is strongly recommended that if a person with autism is told that their family member has committed suicide, specialised counselling help should be sought and made available throughout the bereavement period.

If a bereaved individual lives in a residential service, has a very limited capacity for understanding, and is highly unlikely to find out about, be informed of, or even comprehend the notion of suicide, it is recommended that the cause of death not be mentioned. Should an explanation be necessary, it should be confined to the necessary details, such as 'they took too many pills, which made them fatally ill and the doctor couldn't make them better' (overdose), 'a train ran over them and their body was so hurt and broken that it can't work any more' or 'their body was so hurt and broken, it can't work any more' (hanging).

It cannot be overemphasised that if an individual loses someone close to them by suicide, staff should assess the whole situation carefully.

Much of the above advice applies equally to homicide. Specialist counselling help should be sought if at all possible.

Deciding who will inform other parties of the bereavement

If possible, staff should speak to a person's family and discuss who will take responsibility for telling other people, such as advocates, befrienders, GPs or social workers, about a bereavement (these people's contact details should be kept on a person's file).

All staff members who are likely to come into contact with a bereaved individual should be informed quickly and privately. So that absolute consistency can be maintained in the management of the bereavement, staff should be told of anything significant, such as:

- the relationship of the individual to the deceased, both familial and emotional (whether close and whether contact was frequent, for example)
- if the death was anticipated, whether the individual was aware of this
- the terms in which the death was explained to them, and how they reacted
- whether they will participate in the rituals surrounding death
- previous losses experienced by the person.

You should also decide whether to tell other people who use the service, and in what terms.

Participation in rituals surrounding death

Participating in the rituals surrounding death can help in the grieving process for those without learning disabilities. It provides an opportunity to face the reality of the death, to begin to come to terms with it, to say farewell to the deceased, and to share grief with others. It is now accepted, too, that most people with learning disabilities should be offered the opportunity to participate in bereavement rituals. This is no less true for people with autism. Accordingly, unless a bereaved individual has expressed a clear wish not to participate, staff should be prepared to arrange for them to view the body and attend the funeral or cremation. They should not be excluded because it is thought they would not understand or might be upset.

Make sure that one or two staff members who know the person well accompany them on these occasions so that family members, who may be seriously distressed by their own grief, need not be responsible for them.

If there are good reasons why a person should not participate in some of the rituals, or there are strong objections from the family, these views must be considered.

If a person you support is to be present at any of the rituals surrounding death, make it clear what they should expect. If possible, it may be helpful for staff to gain as much information as they can from family members or religious leaders. It is valuable, if time allows, to visit (or take the person to visit) relevant locations in advance of the funeral – the church, synagogue, temple, mosque, cemetery or crematorium for example. If a person goes to a place of worship regularly, explain that the usual rituals may not occur during a funeral service.
It may help to describe the actions of mourners at a funeral (singing hymns, saying prayers for the deceased, the fact that

the priest or religious leader may speak about the deceased); the meanings of the rituals (as far as they can be understood by the client); and the fact that the body (inside the coffin) will be moved to the front in the ceremony. They should also be told that it is all right to cry at a funeral.

Viewing the body

Viewing a body can help the bereaved to understand the finality of death. If it has been agreed that a person with autism will go to view a body, they should be told what to expect – for example, that it will be cold to touch. Make sure that they know the whole body is there: children, seeing only the head of the deceased in the coffin, have been known to conclude that it has been severed from the body (Schaeffer and Lyons, 1998). It is possible that a person with autism may think this, too. In some instances, therefore, it could be helpful for a person with autism to touch the body.

Avoid viewing a body if it is likely to cause distress. A person with autism may have told you they are reluctant, or your understanding of their temperament may tell you that it is inadvisable. Similarly, if a body has been mutilated in some way, a viewing may not be appropriate.

Funeral

If possible, agree with family beforehand where you will sit or stand during a funeral service. It may be wise to be at the back so that you can make an inconspicuous exit if the person you support becomes too distressed. Point out the coffin and the fact that it is holding the body. If flowers are given, encourage the individual to bring flowers to place on the coffin.

Burial

If a body is to be buried, make it clear that a coffin will protect it from mud and rain. The person you support may wish to join the other mourners in throwing a handful of earth on the coffin.

Cremation

If a body is to be cremated, explain the process and reassure the person you support that the deceased will not feel any pain, as they are no longer able to feel.

Visiting a grave or memorial stone

Even if a person you support has not participated in other rituals, try to arrange a visit to the grave or memorial stone, as this can be a helpful way for them to say goodbye to the deceased. Explain the significance of graves or memorial stones in terms that the person can understand. Perhaps encourage them to make a gesture, such as placing flowers or planting a tree or rose bush. It may be appropriate to arrange further visits, particularly if they are requested. Visits to graves or memorial stones may help with coming to terms with their bereavement. Consideration should be given to whether they could visit it on the anniversary of the death, or on other anniversaries, as a way of remembering the deceased. It is desirable to keep family members informed of these visits, but their permission is not essential.

Memorial services

Some families, particularly if the deceased has been of some prominence in the community, organise a memorial service, usually some weeks after the burial. It may not be appropriate for the person you support to attend the service if a large number of people will be present. However, if the family expresses a wish for them to attend, or if the individual wishes to go, be prepared to explain the significance of the service and to accompany them.

Mementos

One strategy for helping a person you support to come to terms with bereavement, if a close family member has died and home visits are to cease, is to arrange for them to visit the family home and choose objects that are significant for them. They can take these back to the service as mementos; these can help to give a sense of continuity.

Comforting the bereaved

All people with autism have some degree of difficulty with communication and social interaction, and this can make it difficult for staff to discover whether or not grieving is taking place (bearing in mind that grief can be absent or delayed). If you think that a person you support is grieving, make sure that the timing and duration of the grieving process and the 'tasks of mourning' are determined by the bereaved.

You can offer comfort to a bereaved person. Use the forms of communication – verbal, non-verbal or both – that are best understood by them. You can also help by:

- being there when needed
- observing sensitively and understanding when to intervene
- explaining the grieving process in a way that a person understands

- listening to and observing non-verbal expressions of grief
- asking how a person feels and supplying words to help them explain – though be careful not to plant ideas
- talking about the deceased and experiences they shared with the bereaved
- offering emotional support
- offering comfort in ways which the bereaved will accept, for example, physical contact such as touching, holding or massage
- making sure that the bereaved is comfortable and not in physical pain or distress
- if it is compatible with a person's religious and ethnic background, and acceptable to the family, introducing references to after-life belief
- offering reassurance that life's routines will go on and they will continue to be supported
- making sure that the bereaved has a quiet place in which to grieve if they indicate the need.

Facilitating access to therapeutic support

As well as providing comfort and emotional support, the support workers' role is to provide access to therapeutic support which might meet a bereaved person's needs. Seek specialist psychiatric, psychological or therapeutic support if you consider it necessary, but bear in mind that such support can be ineffective and may even be harmful if the practitioner does not have specific knowledge of autism.

Here is a selection of therapeutic approaches:
- counselling
- cognitive behaviour therapy

- social stories
- participation in an appropriate support group
- medication
- opportunities for vigorous exercise
- relaxation techniques
- non-compulsive activities.

These measures can help to alleviate anxiety and depression, conditions which are frequently associated with autism and may be exacerbated by bereavement.

Counselling needs to be carefully planned in advance. This will involve assessment of an individual and their degree of language competence, and the type of language, focus and structure appropriate to the particular circumstances (Tantam, 2000; McCormick, 1998).

Cognitive behaviour therapy, which can help a person to learn strategies for dealing with particular social and emotional problems, requires the expertise of someone who is able to adapt it for people with autism (Attwood, 1998; Prior, 2000).

Social stories are designed to improve understanding of social situations and offer specific behaviour to use when interacting with others (Attwood, 2000; Gray, 1998, 2013). In the context of bereavement, they can be helpful in providing coping strategies and an understanding of other people's reactions to death and grief. Written according to specific guidelines, social stories were initially used mainly with children, but have been successfully adapted for adults.

It is essential, if medication is to be used, that the prescribing doctor is aware of the idiosyncratic reactions of people with autism (Tantam, 2000). You may need to tell doctors about a person's previous reactions to 'drug therapy'.

Facilitating supportive relationships

If a person's parents are no longer alive, staff should be actively involved in facilitating supportive relationships – such as successor parents and citizen advocates – which may have been arranged by the parents. Things like telephone calls, home visits and outings, for which parents were previously responsible, can be very reassuring to a person with autism. In the absence of such relationships, staff may wish to identify people who will reliably perform these functions through organisations such as churches, advocacy or befriending groups. Be sure that the appropriate checks are made and that you introduce the new relationship carefully.

Coping with grief reactions

Staff will wish to take particular note of the common reactions to bereavement listed in Part I so they will have some idea of what a bereaved individual may be feeling. It is helpful to focus on some of these reactions when deciding which kinds of supportive measures are best for a particular person.

Bear in mind that some of these reactions can derive from causes other than bereavement. Familiarity with a person and good powers of observation may help you to determine the cause of any distress, but it is safe to assume that bereavement may be a powerful factor for two years or more after the death of someone close to them.

Anger

If a person you support feels they have been abandoned by someone who has died, they may direct their anger at them. It may also be directed at the person who broke the news of the death, or it may be generalised. You might find that a person gets angry if they can't do activities they used to enjoy with the deceased.

Try to let the person express anger without harming themselves or others, or damaging property. One young man with autism expressed his anger by breaking up the furniture in his room. But it may have been possible to divert his anger into a form of exercise – hitting cushions or a punch bag, knocking a ball about or tearing up old telephone books.

Guilt

Guilt may arise from the 'magical thinking' characteristic of young children who have been bereaved, and who think they might have caused a death by their own actions. Guilt is anger turned on oneself, but in people with autism it is often expressed as overt anger. Avoid suggesting to someone you support that they might have feelings of guilt. However, if it seems that they do, reassure them that the death was inevitable and not caused by their own or anyone else's actions. Be careful to use the same terms in which the death was originally explained.

One young man with Asperger syndrome said that he felt guilty after a death in the family because other family members considered his reactions to be inappropriate. He needed to be reassured that he should not feel guilty, as he had not been aware of how people normally react to bereavement. This was further complicated because he had not been diagnosed at the time and his family were unaware of his need for help and understanding.

Anxiety, fear and panic

Anxiety, fear and panic are all common responses to bereavement. These feelings are likely to be heightened in people with autism, not only because of the loss of someone important in their lives who may have represented stability and security, but also because the changes which almost inevitably follow bereavement are likely to be threatening to a person with autism. The bereavement may also give rise to a fear of their own death, possibly resulting in a fear of going to sleep, or a fear that other members of their family may also die.

It may be helpful to treat anxiety, which can be closely related to depression, with alternatives to medication, such as exercise and relaxation techniques. Severe anxiety can be treated by someone trained in cognitive behaviour therapy (Attwood, 1998), who should also have sufficient knowledge of autism to adapt it accordingly. You can also encourage a successor parent, a befriender or other members of the family to keep in close touch with the person you support. They could, perhaps, fulfil some of the functions previously undertaken by the deceased.

If medication is considered to be necessary, it is essential that the prescribing doctor is which drugs are most appropriate for people with autism (Tantam, 2000; Bogdashina, 2006).

Be prepared to provide constant reassurance and perhaps to take a person out for meals or home visits. Make sure they know that they will still be supported and provide security by maintaining the usual routines of daily life. Unless the person you support has expressed a positive wish for change, do not introduce any changes during the period of bereavement.

Depression and despair

A bereaved person will feel the emptiness and pain of loss acutely, but on no account should staff try to 'jolly' them out of their grief. 'They kept wanting me to dance, but I was too sad to' was a poignant comment made by a bereaved person with learning disabilities (Oswin, 1991).

Talking about the deceased, though it may temporarily exacerbate grief, is considered necessary for recovery from bereavement (Carr, 1988; Todd, 2012). In order to assist this process, learn something about the deceased – how they looked, their personality, the nature of their relationship with the individual, and the activities they shared. Get to know about any terms of endearment the deceased used for the bereaved. This can encourage the person you support to communicate their memories of the deceased, but also help you to speak about the deceased in terms which are meaningful to the person with autism, and from which they may derive comfort. Because people with autism have difficulty in understanding and expressing their feelings, staff need to help them to do this.

It can be difficult to identify depression in a person with autism. Healthcare professionals may unfortunately be unaware of the high risk (McCormick, 1998; Madders, 2010). It is therefore up to service staff to be vigilant in detecting thoughts of suicide and perhaps to introduce therapeutic support. Specialised counselling by people familiar with autism can be helpful, as can participation in an appropriate support group (McCormick, 1998). Psychiatric or psychological intervention may need to be sought for those experiencing prolonged depression. Again, medication should be prescribed only by someone who has a thorough knowledge of the idiosyncratic reactions of people with autism (Tantam, 2000).

Physical symptoms such as pain, appetite disturbance, breathlessness and illness

The physical symptoms of bereavement can cause acute discomfort. It is now generally accepted that bereavement can be responsible for the beginning or exacerbation of genuine illness (Hollins and Sireling, 1999). One young woman with autism who lost her father suffered a serious and prolonged period of asthma combined with anorexia, when she had to be fed by hand. Of course, staff need to determine whether an illness has been triggered by a factor other than bereavement, such as the side-effects of medication. Good food – especially soft food such as yoghurt, soup and puréed foods – and warm drinks can be a source of comfort. Assistance with eating may also be comforting. Body temperature may drop because of bereavement and it may be necessary to make sure that a person is kept warm and comfortable.

Increased need for sleep, sleeplessness and hyperactivity

The bereaved may require more than the usual amount of sleep or, conversely, they may experience insomnia or hyperactivity. Staff will need to balance these reactions with maintaining a stable routine.

Nightmares

Staff on night duty should be made aware not only of the risk of sleeplessness but also of the fact that the bereaved may have frightening and disturbing nightmares. One young woman with autism dreamed she was eating meat, which turned out to be her deceased brother. If the nightmares persist, extra staff may need to be on duty, as the bereaved should be woken up, helped out of bed and given a warm drink. They may need someone to sit with them after they return to bed and while they go to sleep.

Regression and loss of skills

Emotional and physical regression, increased dependency and loss of skills are common reactions to bereavement by people with learning disabilities. They may become uncharacteristically incontinent or bedridden (Hollins and Sireling, 1999; Booklet 3, Cathcart, 1994). Staff should be aware of these possible reactions and it is strongly advised that any assessments should be avoided during a period of bereavement, as it would result in an entirely abnormal reading.

Absence of grief following bereavement

It is now known that some people with autism do not mourn the loss of people close to them. This absence of the grieving process does not appear to be related to a person's cognitive level, nor does it necessarily result in long-term adverse effects. The few examples known to us do not justify an assumption that a person does not have the capacity to feel emotion in another context.

If an individual does not exhibit grief in an expected way, it does not necessarily follow that they are not grieving. Before concluding that an individual is not grieving, staff need to verify their conclusion through careful observation, sensitive questioning and checking the behaviour of the individual in different settings (Tuffrey-Wijne, 2013). Furthermore, it cannot be concluded from the fact that there has not been a reaction to one bereavement that there will be no reaction to subsequent bereavements – particularly the death of a second parent, which may mean home visits stop, and parental support and care is no longer provided.

Problems encountered in bereavement of people with autism

First and foremost, those offering support to a bereaved individual should have a good understanding of autism. But they must also know the person well and be skilled in observing and interpreting both their verbal and non-verbal reactions. The grieving process of people with autism is affected by their difficulties with communication, social interaction and cognition. Staff should be aware of some of the problems that may arise.

Delayed reaction to loss

Grief is often a delayed process for people with learning disabilities. They fail initially to understand the implications of their loss, but may come to feel the impact later (Kitching, 1987). One young woman with autism whose father died before Christmas accepted that she could not go home for the holiday (because Daddy had gone to heaven) but did not begin the grieving process until she went home the following Christmas and realised her father was absent. She then underwent a profound grieving process that lasted for more than two years.

Apparent failure to understand the irreversibility of death

Hollins and Tuffrey-Wijne (2009) suggest that the key issue is not necessarily whether people with communication difficulties understand the irreversibility of death but that professionals give information and answer questions in a way that suits individuals. Adults with autism who have good language skills, a higher than average IQ and who function well in day-to-day-life may want to be kept informed, make their wishes known and most importantly have their preferences honoured (Schuhow and Zurakowski, 2013).

It is normal in the early stages of bereavement to behave as though the deceased is still alive or even present, and to experience difficulty in accepting the finality of death. If a person repeatedly asks about the return of the deceased after a funeral, it can be their way of coming to terms with the loss. They may want to check that everyone gives consistent replies; or the questions may be their way of showing that they need comfort and reassurance. One young man with autism who attended his father's funeral and cremation persisted for some time in asking when his father would return.

Uncertain and inappropriate responses to bereavement

There have been a number of examples of people with autism who have expressed uncertainty about how they should react to the death of someone close to them: 'Should I feel sad?', 'How sad should I feel?', 'Shall I cry?' Others have reacted by giggling at the funeral or at the grave – perhaps a reflection of this uncertainty. Some have appeared callous and unfeeling, which is very difficult for those around them. One girl, following the death of her mother, immediately asked when her father planned to marry again. Some apparently callous comments can be the result of difficulties with verbal expression.

Because people with high-functioning autism and Asperger syndrome can appear to converse normally, they are expected to act like other people too, and reflect conventional emotions. In fact, they may lack the coping mechanisms for dealing with emotions in themselves or others, and can appear to be callous and unfeeling when in fact they are confused, anxious or unable to comprehend the perceptions that others have of them in the event of a bereavement. They may be made to feel that they have done something wrong, yet have no idea of how to put it right. Social stories can be helpful as they provide a 'script' of what will happen and what people say and do in specific circumstances. They can give some insight into how other people are feeling, too. This can alleviate a person's anxiety (Attwood, personal communication, 1999; Giarelli and Gardner, 2012; Handley and Hutchinson, 2012)

Disruptive or challenging behaviour

Because of difficulties with communication and interaction skills, the only way a bereaved person with autism may be able to express their grief is by disruptive or challenging behaviour.

It is difficult for staff to discover whether behaviour arises from fear, anger, anxiety, guilt or physical discomfort – all of which can accompany bereavement – or whether it arises from factors altogether unrelated to bereavement, for example, the effects of medication or distress caused by the behaviour of another person who uses the service. By careful observation and sensitive questioning, if an individual will tolerate it, staff may be able to discover the cause of the behaviour and what a person is trying to communicate. They can then take appropriate action. It may help to encourage a person to participate in an activity which they are known to enjoy, become involved in relaxation (aromatherapy, massage, time in a sensory room), or do exercise such as using gym equipment, jogging or aerobics.

Medication for behavioural problems, particularly aggression, is never an effective long-term solution (Tantam, 2000). It is important to remember that even long after the initial loss, a person's behaviour can be affected by bereavement.

Self-injurious behaviour

Self-injury, which can take the form of head-banging, hand-biting or scratching, arises, like challenging behaviour, from difficulties with communication and interaction. Like challenging behaviour it can signal distress following bereavement, caused by fear, anger or physical discomfort, or it can be used as a means of communication (Attwood, 1993; Sims, 2011). The National Autistic Society has information about self-injury at www.autism.org.uk/challengingbehaviour.

The same measures referred to in the section above (Disruptive or challenging behaviour) can be helpful in discovering the cause of self-injurious behaviour and taking appropriate action, as well as encouraging an individual to participate in an enjoyable activity, a form of relaxation therapy or exercise.

Limited means of expressing grief

It is generally agreed that people without learning disabilities who are bereaved find it helpful to talk to sympathetic family members and friends about the deceased and about their feelings. Grief counselling, proven to have a very positive effect, involves listening to the bereaved and responding reassuringly and supportively. These therapeutic strategies may not be suitable or accessible for everyone with autism, unless staff can help them to express their thoughts and feelings through sensitive questioning and appropriate words, signs or pictures. Because of the demands it makes upon them, this kind of attention may be unwelcome to the bereaved, who may find it threatening. On the other hand, if grief is present and not expressed it may eventually lead to depression or neurosis.

People with autism who are good at conversing may also need help and support to express their reactions to bereavement, which may be complicated by their feelings of inadequacy in responding in the way that others expect. Carefully structured counselling can be an appropriate intervention, as may the use of social stories.

Inability to request help

Some people with autism will be unable or unwilling to seek support when they are anxious, depressed or unhappy. Staff can intervene sensitively.

Limited number of relationships

Many people with autism have comparatively few close relationships. Consequently, there may be a very substantial emotional investment in those relationships and if a person dies, the effects may be catastrophic. Because they have a limited network of family and friends, a person may find it difficult to perform one of the tasks of mourning which must be worked through if the grieving process is to be completed – that is, to find a different place for the deceased in their emotional life and reinvest in new relationships (Worden, 1991).

In common with others with disabilities, many people with autism may be highly dependent for help on professional staff. These staff may not be able to provide long-term emotional support, so it is essential that parents arrange supportive relationships for their son or daughter when they are no longer able to perform these roles, or after they have died (see page 24, Supportive relationships).

Preoccupation with the deaths of people who a person does not know

There are examples of people with autism who are obsessively interested in deaths reported in the media and with whom they have no personal connection. One young man became preoccupied with the death of Diana, Princess of Wales, and a young woman who was obsessively interested in firemen exhibited signs of acute grief on hearing that a firefighter had been killed while trying to rescue someone.

Inability to seek activities which may help the grieving process

People without learning disabilities have a number of strategies which can help to mitigate their loss. They may turn to exercise, pursue their hobbies, seek social contacts, travel or listen to music. People with autism may not have the self-awareness, motivation or experience to seek activities which might be helpful to them, and often will not have access to them unless they are supported by staff, family members or carers.

Introduction of undesirable habits or obsessions

Staff may need to intervene if undesirable habits or obsessions appear during a person's grieving process. They may be a source of comfort at first, but can persist long after the period of grieving, to the detriment of the individual.

Inability to predict future change

People with autism may not understand that the pain and suffering which they are experiencing will eventually come to an end. They therefore lack a possible source of comfort. Staff should make every effort to explain the grieving process to them, bearing in mind that the intensity and duration of their reactions should be determined only. One support worker, when asked by the bereaved, 'Have I finished being sad?' gave her permission for the grieving to finish. She therefore helped the person to resolve her grief (Rawlings, 1996).

Difficulty accepting the need to move on

In the instance of sudden death, because of the intensity of emotions and general trauma of those affected, staff should be especially vigilant in approaching specific areas of sensitivity, for example sorting and dispersing personal possessions and rearranging the deceased's house. A person who has experience the sudden death of a carer or family member may find it hard to come to terms with and move on.

Anniversaries

Many people will need special attention on the anniversary of a death and at specific times of year which they may have celebrated with the deceased, such as Christmas and birthdays.

Grief and growth

The ultimate aim of staff who support people with autism should be to help them resolve their grief, but also to transform their experience into a source of strength for themselves and something that may be of benefit to others. There have been some moving examples of this where people with autism, having experienced bereavement themselves, have offered comfort to other people on the spectrum, or to staff and family members who are bereaved. This is a reminder of the quotation at the start of this book:

"There is no growth without pain and conflict and no loss that cannot lead to gain." (Pincus, 1961)

Part 4: Other aspects of bereavement support

Support for surviving family members

After the death of someone close to a person with autism, particularly a family member, staff may find that they are in close touch with other family members who are also mourning the deceased. Staff should be prepared to offer support to family members in the following ways:

- keeping them informed of the reactions of the person with autism to their loss
- helping family members to understand and come to terms with those reactions, in particular:
  - inappropriate behaviour
  - apparently callous reactions
  - anger, especially if it is directed towards them.

You may find that a person's mother, for example, is the focus of aggression from a bereaved individual, who may hold her responsible for the death. This is especially true if it was the mother who told them about the death. However, family members shouldn't be deterred from visiting because of this. Staff should be prepared to be present and to intervene, if necessary, to protect visitors.

Support for staff caring for a bereaved client

One of the functions of a bereavement support group should be to support staff, too. Caring for a person who has been bereaved can be a very demanding role, requiring great attention and commitment. Staff may find it difficult to determine whether the reactions of the bereaved individual are the result of their grief or related to something else entirely. It can also be distressing to witness another person's grief. The anger that many bereaved people display may be directed towards staff.

Support groups should make sure that staff have access to someone from the group at all times, not only to get advice, but also to get an informed, sympathetic response if they need to talk about their own feelings.

Bereaved staff

Staff who are themselves experiencing the effects of bereavement may wish to seek support from a bereavement support group. Staff might also wish to meet in a 'sharing group' where they can express their feelings about the deceased and their own reactions without fear of interruption or criticism. The sessions might be introduced and led by a senior member of staff, a member of the clergy or a member of Cruse Bereavement Care, who would explain the purpose of the session and how it will be conducted. The sessions should be held in quiet, comfortable surroundings at a pre-arranged time, and should last not more than one hour.

Loss of a client or staff member

For staff in services, the death of a person they support or a colleague can be particularly devastating. The loss may be felt by a number of staff and other people who use the service. In order to cope with losses of this kind, staff need to be prepared to undertake many of the practical arrangements following a death, such as registration and funeral (see part 2, Preparation for bereavement management).

Who to inform

When a person who uses a service dies, anyone who is likely to be affected should be told – including staff. Remember that other people with autism may detect differences in people's moods or the general feeling of the service. They can misapprehend the reasons for this change, and this misapprehension may cause more distress than the truth. Whether people should be informed as a group or individually depends on their relationship to the deceased and to each other. People's families should also be told, in case they need to offer extra support to their relatives.

Support for other people who use the service

It is important to identify people using a service who are likely to grieve for the deceased. You can appoint a bereavement support worker who can help people through the grieving process and enable them take part in the rituals surrounding death, such as funerals or cremations.

Support for surviving family members

Staff may find that they are called upon to offer support to family members of a deceased person, especially if they are parents. Autism, by its very nature, can isolate a person from others. Family members may therefore turn to staff, being perhaps some of the few people who knew and liked their relative as an individual, and who were sympathetic to their needs. One part of the grieving process is the need to talk about the deceased. Staff are uniquely qualified to listen sympathetically to family members and help them come to terms with their loss.

Support for survivors of suicide

If a person takes their own life, both staff and family members can find this particularly difficult to come to terms with and may need expert counselling. The book *A Special Scar*, by Alison Wertheimer, is helpful in explaining the experience of people bereaved by suicide (see References).

Memorial services or ceremonies

The opportunity to say goodbye can be important when people are grieving. A memorial service, which those who knew a person can help to organise and in which they can participate, can help in this respect. It is also a way to recall the life of the deceased in a positive way. Local religious or secular figures can be asked to officiate and to advise on the form the service might take. Alternatively, or in addition, a ceremony such as installing a bench, planting a tree or erecting a memorial stone can be beneficial.

If people who use services are to attend a funeral or memorial service, they should not go out in a minibus as if on an outing. Despite the expense, care should be taken to arrive in a more respectful and appropriate manner (Oswin, 1991).

Part 5: Support for the dying

Care of the dying

Palliative care refers to the type of care given to patients whose disease is not responsive to curative treatment. Control of pain, of other symptoms and of psychological, social and spiritual problems is paramount. The goal of palliative care is the achievement of the best quality of life for patients and their families (SMAC, 1992).

There are three groups of people who are likely to be involved in palliative care of the dying:

- support staff employed by a service that the person uses
- healthcare professionals, in particular nursing staff
- the family of the patient.

If the relationship of these groups to each other is based on co-operation, mutual respect and good communication, this will have a positive impact on the quality of palliative care which they can deliver to a patient (Read, 1998).

Training for support staff

As part of bereavement training in services for adults with autism, it is recommended that at least some staff should be trained in support for the dying, including the principles of palliative care. The website of Help the Hospices offers a great deal of relevant and up-to-date information and details of useful organisations (see Useful contacts). As with bereavement support, the approach you take to care for the dying will be different for each individual, but certain principles apply to everyone.

The needs of support staff

It is important to make sure that the needs of support staff in the service that a person normally uses are adequately met. For example, staff may require:

- counselling or psychological support so that they can, in turn, help a person with autism to manage their feelings of fear and anxiety
- support with the process of breaking bad news in a way that is understandable to a person with autism
- advice on communicating with a person in a way that will minimise the risk of causing anxiety
- help to get information about the needs of a person with autism and the course of their illness (Read, 1998).

Knowing the individual patient well

Preferably, a small number of key support staff will be dedicated to the care of a dying person, and, if at all possible, serve in this capacity until death. These staff members should know the patient well, so the client has complete confidence in them, and so that they can interpret the person's verbal and non-verbal reactions to make sure they receive the care they need. Many people with autism will not openly indicate when they are feeling pain or discomfort. Support staff must therefore be observant, so that they can alleviate a person's anxiety and discomfort and advocate on their behalf to healthcare professionals.

Communication: the need for tranquillity and a consistent approach

If a person is receiving palliative care, it is vital that they do not become anxious, and that their mental tranquility is maintained at all times, if at all possible. This can be achieved by making sure that care and communication is consistent.

Support staff

Staff should communicate effectively with each other every day, both about the care provided to a person and what is said to them. Uncertainty or inconsistency on the part of support staff can be easily picked up by a person with autism, leading to anxiety.

Healthcare professionals

Support staff will need to act as mediators between healthcare professionals and people with autism to make sure that they can communicate well, and that consistent information is given in a way that is accessible to individuals.

Family and friends

Every effort should be made to make sure that family members and friends who visit people with autism are in agreement with each other and with staff on the type of support that should be provided, and the information that should be given to the person about their illness.

Communication with the patient: the need for tact and care

The issue of how much information should be given to a dying person with autism can be determined only by a careful assessment of each individual, and consultation with support staff and family members who wish to be involved. It is important that everyone concentrates on providing reassurance and quality of life to the dying, one day at a time – bearing in mind the need to avoid anxiety.

Staff should learn about the symptoms and the expected course of an illness, communicating this information only if there are positive reasons for doing so (for example, failure to provide answers to persistent questions from a patient will cause increased anxiety).

For many people with autism who appear to have limited communication and understanding, it might seem that providing information about the progression and outcome of their illness would be in their best interests. Although the person may have some understanding of death, they may not be able to grasp that it is happening to them. Probing to find out about the person's perception of death may serve only to arouse their anxieties. However, support staff and their managers need to be aware of their responsibilities under the *Mental Capacity Act 2005* (England and Wales) and *Adults with Incapacity (Scotland) Act 2000*. In some cases it might be deemed necessary to use an autism-experienced advocate to attempt to ascertain a person's wishes (Parsons and Sims, 2010). To find a local advocate visit www.actionforadvocacy.org.uk.

There are numerous resources related to death and bereavement for support staff working with people with a learning disability. The Palliative Care for People with Learning Disabilities Network website has useful information about the best and most relevant resources to choose (www.pcpld.org/links-and-resources). However, when communicating information to people with autism, staff should make a judgement based on their assessment of a person's understanding of their illness and its implications for their own death. A person may need help and support to explore their feelings about dying, death and after-life beliefs. Support staff must take the lead from the person with autism, while at the same time avoiding false hopes.

People with autism have difficulty accepting changes in routine, and dealing with uncertainty in their futures. Support staff who know a person well can use coping strategies which have previously been successful, to help maintain their peace of mind.

Some people with autism can, at times, simultaneously hold two incompatible ideas in their minds, a condition which has been observed in people facing the prospect of death (Lansdown, 1996). Denial may also be a means of coping with the prospect of death.

It is strongly recommended that staff, especially those supporting people with a high level of comprehension, read Part 3 of the book *Death, Dying and Bereavement* (edited by Dickenson and Johnson, 1993) called 'Caring for Dying People'. This details strategies for dealing with uncertainty, denial and difficult questions raised by the dying.

The religious dimension

If a person with autism is associated with a religious community or holds particular beliefs, support staff should seek advice from relevant people in that community about the rituals of dying and death. Most clergy are accustomed to supporting the dying and they could help to support a person if they are carefully briefed about their autism and its effects. Again, it is strongly recommended that staff read the relevant chapters in *Death, Dying and Bereavement* (mentioned above). *Death and Bereavement Across Cultures* (edited by Parkes et al, 1997) is also a useful book.

The patient's physical comfort

Paying attention to a person's physical comfort includes not only pain control but also making sure that, for example, their bed and sheets are comfortable and clean, that blankets are used so that the 'weighting' can be varied as necessary, and that the room temperature and ventilation are well-maintained and suit the person. Consideration should be given to the use of complementary therapies which can help to induce relaxation, such as massage and aromatherapy.

Appropriate diet

It is important that a person with autism follows a diet appropriate to their appetite and healthcare needs, having regard not only to taste but also to consistency. Support staff may need to help a person to eat by encouraging them or by actually feeding them. This is particularly necessary in a hospital environment in case people who cannot feed themselves miss out.

Location

If possible, a dying person should be cared for in familiar, quiet and tranquil surroundings. Ideally, this should be in their home. If a person shares their home with other people with autism, appropriate support and information should be given to those people, too.

If care in a hospice is considered appropriate, or if the appropriate level of care can only be maintained by keeping a person in hospital, arrangements should be made for service staff who know the dying person well to provide 24-hour cover if possible. This allows staff to communicate between the person and healthcare professionals and to advocate on their behalf.

Access to palliative care

People with autism should, if they need it, have access to palliative care services, which include nursing care, pain control and symptom management. Referral to these services is usually arranged by a consultant, GP or district nurse. Palliative care can be provided in a hospice, a hospital, or a person's home. It can take the form of nursing care or advice (given to those carrying out day-to-day care for a person with autism). Individual care plans should be developed which may include pain relief, pressure care, physiotherapy, family support, the religious dimension and day services (Murdy and O'Leary, 1999). If a person uses day services, the plan may include Snoezelen sessions (time in a sensory room) and therapeutic activities that the person is known to enjoy.

Help the Hospices' Intelligence Hub (www.helpthehospices.org.uk/our-services/intelligence-hub/) publishes a directory listing all palliative care services in the UK and Republic of Ireland.

Cancer care

For people with cancer, palliative care expertise can be provided through the NHS by Macmillan Cancer Support and Marie Curie Cancer Care – both charitable bodies – by a referral from a patient's GP or district nurse. District nurses, contacted through GPs, are responsible for assessing patients' nursing requirements.

Macmillan nurses, who work in hospitals and in the community, advise on pain control and symptom management, give guidance on treatments available and offer psychological and emotional support to patients and those who support them.

Marie Curie nurses give practical nursing care to patients throughout the day, overnight in their own homes or in Marie Curie centres. They can also support a limited number of people with life-shortening illnesses other than cancer. The practical work of Marie Curie nurses complements that of Macmillan nurses, whose role is mainly advisory. In some cases, depending upon their needs, patients benefit from both types of nursing.

Issues relating to palliative care for people with learning disabilities

As people with learning disabilities and complex needs have the right to live in the community, most people with autism now depend on primary healthcare teams to meet their medical needs.

Several studies have shown that the medical needs of many people with learning disabilities have been overlooked, delaying access to palliative care (Tuffrey-Wijne, 2013; Heslop et al, 2013). Various causes have been identified, including:

- communication impairment on the part of people with learning disabilities
- failure of health professionals, carers or support staff to recognise symptoms of pain and illness
- health professionals, carers or support staff mistakenly attributing symptoms to a person's learning disability rather than to a physical illness
- lack of healthcare screening generally available to the wider population.

Some suggested recommendations for overcoming this issue are:

- improved awareness by carers and support staff of the signs and symptoms of early stages of diseases
- increased awareness of learning disability on the part of healthcare professionals
- improvement in healthcare screening (Tuffrey-Wijne, 1997).

In 1998, the National Network for the Palliative Care of People with Learning Disabilities was formed. It is now called the Palliative Care for People with Learning Disabilities (PCPLD) Network and it promotes access to palliative care for people with learning disabilities. Among its aims are:

- to identify and promote good practice
- to provide information, training and research
- to highlight the need for ease of access for people with learning disabilities to mainstream palliative care services and the related need for the creation of some specialist learning disability care services.

Two groups of people with learning disabilities have been identified who are most in need of specialist palliative care services:

- those with profound disabilities who are unable to use verbal communication
- those with challenging behaviour (Murdy and O'Leary, 1999).

Relevance to people with autism

Issues relating to palliative care for people with learning disabilities are relevant to people with autism. The autism spectrum includes a significant number of people who fall into the two groups for whom mainstream palliative care services are not considered appropriate – those with a severe communication condition and those perceived to have challenging behaviour. These groups of people would need specialist palliative care services, whether in a hospice, a hospital or at home.

However, the needs of many people with autism are so complex that even if they do not have learning disabilities or complex needs, specialised palliative care services might have to be devised for them. Support staff could help to do this by working in co-operation with specialist teams.

Commitment to the dying

Among staff who have demonstrated a strong commitment to providing the best possible quality of life to each person with autism in their care, it is to be hoped that there are some who, when called upon to do so, will demonstrate an equally strong commitment to ensuring as dignified and as peaceful death as possible.

Acknowledgements

Sincere thanks are owed to all those who gave valuable help and support during the preparation of this work and its revisions.

Those who were kind enough to contribute their experiences of supporting bereaved people with autism have been acknowledged in the introduction to the Appendices. Particular mention has been made of the valuable contribution by the young man with Asperger syndrome who described his own experiences of bereavement.

Appendices

Appendix I was compiled from the results of a survey undertaken for the paper *The management of bereavement in services for people with autism*, published in 1992. A total of 20 respondents to a notice in The National Autistic Society members' magazine, among whom were both parents and care staff, completed a questionnaire on individuals with autism whom they had supported during their grieving process. Ten responses which were considered to represent the breadth of the spectrum are included in this appendix. It is likely that several of these people would now be diagnosed as having Asperger syndrome. One of the two additional contributions received from parents who did not complete the questionnaire referred to their family member as having Asperger syndrome.

Appendix II resulted from a request to those who supported people with Asperger syndrome through the grieving process. Only two responses were received, one from parents and one from care staff. In addition, a young man with Asperger syndrome offered a very moving account of his bereavement experience.

A particular debt of gratitude is owed to the relatives who helped with this study, and to the young man with Asperger syndrome, as in so doing they were reliving their own experiences of bereavement.

All of the contributions have been valuable, both in providing background information for this book and in validating its recommendations. They demonstrate how sensitive management can help bereaved people with autism towards a successful resolution of grief.

The names of the bereaved have been changed in order to preserve confidentiality.

Appendix I: Grief reactions of people with autism

Alan

Age at time of bereavement: 14.

Description: highly dependent, needing constant supervision and frequent physical intervention. Able to converse and express preferences and feelings; some ritualistic behaviour; a high level of anxiety; hyperactive; mood swings; epileptic. In residential school: termly boarding at time of bereavement.

Relationship to deceased: grandmother; close and affectionate.

How was bereaved told of death? Mother told him, 'Nana was very ill, so Jesus invited her to his wonderful garden. She is happy now and wants you to know she will always love you.'

Immediate reactions: ran round the room with grief. Then cuddled by his mother and cried on her shoulder. He said, 'Mummy, I do love you,' then, 'Nana, oh my Nana.' Shock then set in and he did not speak for three days.

Later reactions: epileptic attacks; temperature; lethargy; depression; disinterested in food and drink; stomach upset. He said he was sad and frightened and was unresponsive. Concerned about mother's health. Tried to hurry past end of road where grandmother lived and did not wish to visit her house again.

Funeral and rituals: did not attend funeral. Took flowers to the crematorium garden but refused to visit ever again. Will not look towards it when he passes.

Support: warm support from mother. Assurance that Nana did not 'go away' and that he could talk about his sadness. Demonstrations of caring and affection (physical contact).

Resolution of grief: happy to have his grandmother's radio, a clock and some of her pictures. Speaks of her often: 'Nana liked those autumn tints', 'Is Nana pleased with me?'

Derek

Age at time of bereavement: 17.

Description: dependent and needing constant supervision. Speech very limited but can express preferences and feelings. Usually cheerful but sometimes sad or worried. Occasional challenging behaviour when feeling insecure. Some periods of anxiety. Termly boarder at school at time of bereavement.

Relationship to deceased: father; close and affectionate.

How was bereaved told of death? His mother told him, 'Daddy is in heaven.'

Type of death: death was anticipated but bereaved did not know of illness.

Immediate reactions: disbelief. He asked, 'Where is Daddy?' and was told, 'In heaven.' Afterwards he did not comment.

Later reactions: no indication of awareness of loss. Asked again, 'Where is Daddy?'

Funeral and rituals: did not participate in any bereavement rituals.

Support: staff at school and his mother who arranged for the bereaved to have frequent home visits and who ensured that he was aware of her affection for him.

Resolution of grief: difficult to detect as no apparent grieving process.

Subsequent bereavements: grandfather died five years later. He was told, 'Grandad is in heaven', and appeared undisturbed. He never asked about him again. The family dog died nine years after his father. The bereaved was told, 'Kelly is in heaven with Daddy and Grandad.' He continues to speak of him as though he were alive, eg 'Take Kelly for a walk.'

Comments: mother is concerned about the effect of her own death on her son and is pleased that her sister and elder son make a practice of arranging for him to visit them, particularly when she is on holiday.

Donald

Age at time of bereavement: 29.

Description: dependent and needing constant supervision in living and working. Very articulate. Normally stable, but anxiety caused by unexpected events, and challenging behaviour only when disturbed. Very much concerned about world events eg nuclear threat, world ecology. Living at home and a day patient at an industrial therapy unit at the time of bereavement.

Relationship to deceased: brother; close and affectionate.

How was bereaved told of death? At the time of death he was on holiday at a Steiner community familiar to him because he had frequently spent periods of time there. As he had attended Steiner schools before, he accepted their religious beliefs, including a firm belief in an after-life. Death was explained in these terms.

Type of death: death was sudden.

Immediate reactions: no particular changes in behaviour but a great need to talk about the deceased and the effect of the loss on his own life as deceased really cared about him. Read his obituaries, looked at photographs, looked at slides the deceased had sent him.

Funerals and rituals: bereaved away from home and did not attend funeral.

Support: staff well-known to him helped him through the first few weeks with excellent counselling. He was able to speak about his loss.

Later reactions: talks about death frequently. He has signed a consent form for his brain to be used for research after death. Anticipates that parents, in their 70s, will die soon. It is predicted that when his mother dies his behaviour will become very disturbed, if not violent. He realises that her death could mean loss of the family home. Talks of committing suicide when both parents are dead (previously, when depressed, made an attempt). Hopes he will not live to old age.

Religious beliefs: greatly influenced by Steiner philosophy. Firm belief in an after-life in which he will have no disability and in which he will be able to do all the things he has not been able to do in this life.

Comments: for ten years the anniversary of his brother's death was marked by rituals of reading his obituaries, looking at photographs and at slides sent to him by the deceased. On the tenth anniversary, he said this would be the last one to be marked by the usual ceremonies and that he could not go on mourning forever.

Dorothy

Age at time of bereavement: 37.

Description: dependent but requiring supervision in living and working and, with occasional physical intervention, able to express preferences and to converse. Occasional speech, occasional anxiety, ritualistic and obsessive when distressed, passive, equable with occasional anger, unable to express feelings. In residential care at time of bereavement.

Relationship to deceased: father; close and affectionate. Home visits (one or two weeks) four times a year. Postal contact every fortnight.

How was bereaved told of death? Two members of staff. The one responsible for bereavement support spoke and the other was unobtrusively present to observe reactions. Death was explained in the same terms as that of her mother, who had died three years previously. She was told, 'Daddy's pain has stopped, he has died and is in heaven with Mummy. The cat is being cared for by neighbours.'

Type of death: the bereaved knew that her father was ill. She had not gone home for the summer holiday.

Immediate reactions: client apparently understood the loss immediately. She said 'Daddy'. She went very quiet and was later heard talking in the accent she uses when re-living early memories.

Later reactions: subdued for several days. On being questioned by another resident about her forthcoming holiday she said, 'I am not going home because Daddy has gone to heaven,' without appearing upset. Showed signs of impatience when things could not be done immediately and less talkative with staff. General irritability.

Funerals and rituals: attended funeral accompanied by two staff members. She did not join in with the singing as she would normally, but no other unusual reactions. Present at cremation and committal. The service meant very little to her and she did not ask about the coffin. She visited the family home and very much enjoyed talking with relatives and guests. Her brother sorted out records and mementoes for her to keep. On leaving she said, 'Dad wasn't home today.' She seemed to accept the reminder that Daddy was in heaven with Mummy. On the way home she was heard to say, 'When Dad's back from heaven, I will go home on the coach.'

Support: mature staff member who accompanied her to the funeral and was regularly available and on call if not on duty.

Long-term reactions: questionnaire completed before these could be determined. It is believed that the previous bereavement had given the client some understanding of death. It has been observed that she interacts more with staff and other clients than she did before her bereavement.

Elizabeth

Age at time of bereavement: 20.

Description: dependent and needing supervision in living and working. Communicates with ease and able to converse; suffers episodes of anxiety which can be resolved if reason is known; frequently obsessive and ritualistic; pinches herself; challenging behaviour in response to certain words, objects, music and also the death of her brother; very high mathematical ability – 'savant', and also artistic. In residential care at time of bereavement.

Relationship to deceased: brother; close and affectionate.

How was bereaved told of death? Stepmother explained that her brother had been taken up to heaven because he had been 'poorly' and also had a sore leg. He was no longer in pain and was happy now.

Immediate reactions: she wanted to know when it happened and at what time. She was angry because her brother had left her.

Later reactions: it was one week before she cried and realised she would not see her brother again. When contact with him would normally have occurred – she had gone home every weekend and for holidays – she became depressed, aggressive, tore clothes and self-harmed. Her sleeping pattern changed and she became destructive. She was prescribed medication for severe depression. Also complained of headaches, stomach pains and a very sad feeling in her heart, and fears of her own death. Suffered a nightmare centred on her brother, a 'black hole in the ground' [grave]. Questions centred on the 'black hole in the ground.' She dreamed that her father was forcing her to eat meat which was her brother's flesh. She asked questions about heaven and spoke of hearse, coffin and graves.

Funeral and rituals: the family considered it unwise for her to attend.

Support: senior care worker who was available to counsel, listen and comfort and who talked to her, explaining that heaven was a wonderful place. She asked her to look at the sky and see how peaceful it looked and told her it was good to cry. She took her to church to light candles on her brother's birthday and 'talk' to him.

Comments: bereaved has been able to offer reassurance to a client whose grandmother died and also to a bereaved member of staff.

Frederick

Age at time of bereavement: 20.

Description: moderately able and can live and work with partial autonomy. Problems of motivation; able to converse; ritualistic in small things; anxious if routine is disturbed; verbal abuse if anxiety is acute; otherwise, equable and passive. Living at home and holding an independent job in the community at time of bereavement.

Relationship to deceased: father; emotionally distant.

Previous bereavement: lost grandfather whom he loved. Spoke about him: 'Would Grandad have been at the cricket match?'

How was bereaved told of death? Mother said, 'Daddy had a heart attack and the doctors could not help him to get well, so God took him to heaven to make him better.'

Type of death: death was sudden.

Immediate reactions: no emotion. He put soup spoon down and said, 'Are you all right, Mum?', 'Why can't Charles [foster brother] come home and be head of this family?', 'I don't want a stepfather.' Understood loss immediately and reacted by fulfilling father's tasks such as coal carrying, walking the dog and cleaning the car.

Later reactions: followed normal routines. Watched father's cricket team as usual, sitting at tea with the cricketers as though father was still present. Blinked back tears when looking at father's photograph. Accepted mother changing her seat at the table (taking father's chair). This was surprising as he is normally fiercely resistant to change. Took mother's hand when going to church a week after father's death when normally he would not have walked with her. Became more responsive to mother, helping with household tasks not previously undertaken, such as cutting the grass. Did not express grief verbally. After one year took a keen interest in mother's male friends, expressing regret if relationship broke down.

Funeral and rituals: present at funeral and cremation. Smiled at congregation as he passed them.

Support: a close male friend of his mother and father took over some of father's caring role such as taking him to football matches and buying him an electric razor.

Resolution of grief: mother has tried to encourage him to speak of father but without success. He continually looks at family photographs, including those of early childhood. Has totally accepted his step-father. He tells him, 'I will call you Dad when you marry Mum.'

Comments: duration of grieving process two years. Support of father's friend in ensuring continuity of normal activities.

Harriet

Age at time of bereavement: 34.

Description: dependent and requiring supervision in living and working. Very limited language but able to express preferences; able to express thoughts and feelings in writing, but only with mother; high level of anxiety and many fears (death, wars, natural disasters, accidents to parents). Usually reassurance and diversion can ensure she is settled and happy, but occasionally nothing can alleviate her anxiety, in which case challenging and compulsive behaviour can result. In residential care at time of bereavement.

Relationship to deceased: grandfather; close and affectionate. Saw him most days when she lived at home. After she went to residential care, he stayed at the family home during her visits.

How was bereaved told of death? Key worker told her that Grandpa had died peacefully: he was not ill but very old. Three months before the death, her mother had broken her hip when Harriet was on a home visit. On return to residential care she lost weight and exhibited challenging behaviour. Staff and her parents agreed to delay telling her of grandfather's death until after she had seen her mother walking normally again and her behaviour had settled.

Type of death: death was anticipated. She appeared to realise that her grandfather was failing well before he died. He was unable to visit the family home during one holiday and on her return staff noticed disturbed behaviour. Staff believed this resulted from a change in medication but her parents were convinced it was her awareness of impending loss.

Immediate reaction: accepted news calmly.

Later reaction: when parents visited, they noticed she had scratches on her hands and face. There were tears when grandfather was mentioned and she appeared grief-stricken. Later she wrote, 'We are sad to think of Grandpa in his coffin.' Many times she said that he was in his house and would come back.

Funeral and rituals: because of distance and necessary delay in telling client of the death, she did not attend the funeral.

Support: very caring key worker who gave her extra attention.

She shrank from physical contact.

Previous bereavements: grandmother died 13 years previously and client reacted with some disturbance. Two other deaths known to her. All deaths increase her anxiety about her own parents' deaths.

Resolution of grief: later she wrote that she knew the happy times with Grandpa would not return but that she remembered them.

Duration of grieving process: six months before death and six months after it.

Religious beliefs: influenced by attendance at Steiner School and Christian beliefs. Parents have explained that we meet our loved ones in the after-life.

Larry

Age at time of bereavement: 3 (age when questionnaire completed: 20).

Description: highly dependent and needing constant supervision and frequent physical intervention. Able to speak with difficulty; bangs his head to force words out (not yet able to speak at time of bereavement). Panic attacks; obsessive; collecting objects which others would discard; self-harm.

Relationship to deceased: grandfather; close and affectionate.

Lived in the same house.

How was bereaved told of death? Mother said, 'Grandad has died and is not in pain any more.'

Type of death: death was anticipated. Larry was aware that his grandfather was in hospital during the fortnight before his death.

Immediate reactions: screamed on the evening of funeral. Not long after funeral he was humming parts of Beethoven's Ninth Symphony, one of his grandfather's favourites.

Later reactions: screaming at bed-time – his grandfather used to play violin and sing to him at bed-time; humming Beethoven; appeared to be in pain; prone to infections, anxiety and hyperactivity.

Funerals and rituals: not present at funeral but was taken to the burial by a neighbour. On later occasions helped to tidy the grave and waved goodbye.

Resolution of grief: bereaved used to speak of 'Grandad at the cemetery' but now no longer mentions him.

Anniversary of death: anxiety around the time of the anniversary of death, but this was also the date of Larry's first visit to the hospital residence where he now resides.

Long-term reactions: wanting to die/afraid of dying.

Comments: mother describes Larry's life as a series of bereavements: losing his grandfather at the age of three; sent by local authority to weekly boarding school 25 miles from his home at age seven; losing father through failure of parents' marriage; admitted to permanent residence in hospital at age 12. He is not allowed to visit home as staff say that he is 'too attached' to it, nor is his grandmother, of whom he is fond, allowed to visit him. He cannot listen to Beethoven's Ninth Symphony as it makes him feel 'too sad.'

Malcolm

Age at time of bereavement: 28 (father), 31 (mother).

Description: moderately able and can live and work with partial autonomy. Extremely chatty; high and frequent anxiety; obsessional, especially about antiques and china; relates well to elderly females; occasionally depressed, but changeable moods; passive, tendency to laziness. In at the time of bereavement.

Relationship to deceased: ambivalent towards father; close and affectionate with mother.

Type of death: in both cases the bereaved knew they were ill.

Immediate reactions when told of deaths: disbelief with father, anxious about him not really being dead, saying, 'Promise me he is really dead.' Soon afterwards he sought reassurance about his mother's health. When told of his mother's death, he said, 'Oh really?' It took two or three days for him to realise that he had suffered a loss. He then said, 'I miss her.'

Later reactions: could talk about his father's death. Of his mother he said, 'I miss her.' After her death he became very dependent on staff. There was a marked increase in anxiety with related hyper-ventilation. He frequently expressed a sense of loss, particularly about home visits and being spoiled by his mother. He became very withdrawn on the first Mother's Day after his mother's death when he realised there was no point in sending a card.

Funeral and rituals: understood significance of rituals. Father's funeral was a 'social event' for the bereaved where he exhibited no sense of loss. He attended mother's funeral, brought flowers and laid them on the coffin. He was very involved and expressed sadness at each stage, though he did not weep. He was able to share his feelings with other, older relatives.

Support: mother after father's death and principal of residential service after mother's death. Encouraged to talk about the deceased; efforts made to ensure that staff were available to offer support.

Resolution of grief: adjusted to loss of his father in less than a year. As the questionnaire was completed soon after the death of his mother, it is difficult to reach conclusions about resolution of grief. He still says, 'I miss her' and 'I haven't anywhere to go now.'

Matthew

Age at time of bereavement: 31.

Description: moderately able and capable of partial autonomous living and working. He is able to express feelings and converse easily, but rarely initiates conversation. He will always try to steer conversations in the direction of his own interests, eg to past personalities in his own life or 1960s and 70s celebrities. Suffers from anxiety deriving from overhearing conversations which he assumes are about himself. Exhibits rare challenging behaviour directed at his mother or people who remind him of her. Lack of confidence, cheerful at times, moody at others. In residential care at the time of bereavement.

Relationship to deceased: father; ambivalent.

How was the bereaved told of death? Client cannot remember and relevant staff member has departed.

Immediate reactions: very matter-of-fact.

Later reactions: effects of bereavement unclear to staff. Bereaved is very matter of fact, referring to the deceased as 'my late father who's dead now.'

Funeral and ritual: bereaved did not attend funeral on grounds that it would be too difficult for his mother. At the express request of his mother, the bereaved has not been permitted to visit the memorial stone. The client has acquiesced, not wishing to upset his mother.

Resolution of grief: no reference is made to the deceased by client. If someone else initiates the subject, he refers to the deceased as 'my late father who's dead now.'

Additional contributions

Thirteen-year-old boy with Asperger syndrome: parents were separated but the father maintained close contact with the boy. The father died suddenly and the boy returned to school on the following Monday, telling staff that 'two sad things had happened' the previous Saturday: his father had died and Crystal Palace had lost their football match. Since then he has spoken about his father's death in a very matter-of-fact way, with no apparent awareness of any emotional implications.

Sixteen-year-old girl with autism and severe epilepsy: when the bereavement occurred she was living in residential school. Her father died suddenly and her mother came to the school to inform her. She replied 'That's nice that daddy's gone to heaven.' Later, when shopping with her mother, she said, 'Oh, that's sad. You won't have to buy daddy's tea now.'

Appendix II: Grief reactions of people with Asperger syndrome

Alfred

Age at time of bereavement: 24.

Description: low independence skills; prone to high anxiety; very moody; social interactions are active but odd. In residential care, visiting home every third weekend.

Relationship to deceased: grandmother; close and affectionate.

How was bereaved told of death? Parents explained, 'Nanny has died.'

Type of death: death was sudden.

Immediate reactions: quiet but calm.

Later reactions: he had many upsets at the residential home, but was deemed to be depressed and put on medication. The parents believed that he was exhibiting a normal grief reaction and that medication was ill-advised. Parents behaved very naturally with him, speaking of his grandmother frequently and recalling the good times they had together. They lit candles in churches with him.

Funeral and rituals: attended cremation but didn't really understand how to react. He was very supportive to his cousins who were visibly upset.

Support: lighting candles in memory of the deceased, talking with parents, extended family and staff.

Previous bereavement: close family friend, aunt, grandfather, grandmother, uncle, teacher.

Resolution of grief: about nine to 12 months, but when anxious will refer to all the people close to him who have died.

Alice

Age at time of bereavement: not given, but in an adult service.

Description: fearful that her new placement might not be permanent; anxious; suffering from low self-esteem; history of anorexia and bulimia (her deceased friend also had anorexia). At the time of bereavement, in a residential service for people with Asperger syndrome to which she had recently been transferred.

Relationship to deceased: female friend who was a resident in the service from which Alice had recently transferred.

How was bereaved told of death? Staff told her of the death.

Type of death: death was by suicide.

Immediate reactions: she was told of the death on the same day she had a review of her new placement. The staff were unable to tell whether the anxiety she exhibited arose from her fear that her new placement might not be permanent or from the news of her friend's death.

Later reaction: a few weeks after hearing of her friend's death, she heard on the news that a fireman had been killed in the course of his duties and exhibited acute grief reactions. She showed more signs of grief over this man than at any time after her friend's death. She is obsessed with firefighters and the fire service.

Support: the staff of the service caring for her. They were aware that she might need support on the anniversary of her friend's death or the date of her friend's birthday.

George

Age at time of report: 31 (had recently been diagnosed as having Asperger syndrome).

In response to his request, he was sent the paper *The management of bereavement in services for people with autism* (1992). He then wrote a letter, from which the following are extracts.

'I had never thought about [bereavement]. Even though I have been to a few funerals, nothing ever stirred in me. I was just following everyone else and mimicking them. When I read through [the paper] I went into a state of shock. I was angry and confused… Then slowly I started to have… insights into some feelings and thoughts I have been trying to work out for years. 'I was overwhelmed with guilt and have been for a long time, 17 years at least. I [realised that] I had felt guilt because of my dog's death.

'When I was about 13-14 years, old my dog was old and dying…

I was playing by myself as usual when I put my leg through a piece of glass. Suddenly my dog bit me and pulled me over. I kicked out and shouted at him. This is what I have felt guilty about. (Shortly afterwards the dog was put down).

'My dog was the only friend I ever had... I constantly got things wrong and was punished by my parents. I was safe with him, sitting next to him and feeling his soft brown coat. I think my dog was my only real source of giving and receiving love. I have cried about my dog as visions of him have entered my mind. I am beginning to realise that my family interaction was and still is distant. I am realising that I had some sort of love for my dog, a love which I find hard to understand with other people

'My dog died when I was 13 years of age. At the time I felt nothing. I was told he had gone but this had no meaning for me. This is the time I started to feel bad about my behaviour and a self-consciousness was forming, but all I knew is that I was told I was bad and so thought I was bad.

'When I was 21 years of age my favourite auntie died. This was the first funeral ritual that I attended. I was just following and mimicking everyone else. I never really understood why people were crying and I didn't express any emotion... A year later another auntie died. I attended this funeral but again nothing stirred in me. When I was 27 years of age my mother's boyfriend died. Again I went to the funeral and acted out the emotions of others.'

There were a number of other bereavements, starting from when he was four years of age, when he was left in the back of a car on his own during his grandmother's funeral. Later ones included the death of his grandfather, a friend from nursery school and an uncle (not known about at the time) and the death of a pet mouse.

'Out of all these issues of bereavement, I have trouble feeling or responding to them, expect for one, my dog Ringo... This is the only one that means anything to me and the only one where I can express real tears and emotion. One of the problems I have with emotions and feelings is that this concept is new to me, for it is only in the last four years that I have understood that this concept exists and is natural. I am still trying to understand feelings and how they interact with the rest of me. Self-awareness is something I have to learn about... Even though in my mind I know that people die, this means nothing to me. I suppose the semantic pragmatics of death and the difficulty I have in understanding this is like my problem with understanding interpersonal relationships and concepts like that of God.

'But what is confusing is this feeling of guilt that I have identified with my dog, for it is the same feeling that in reflection I was made to feel by my parents and the schools because of how I behaved... It is the feeling that controlled me and my 'bad' behaviour. It's the feeling that triggered my intelligence to mimic and pretend to interact, even though I never knew why.

'The only extrapolation I can make is an intellectual one, where I have learnt that society and religion use the process of guilt as a form of control and that, perhaps due to my dog's death, I have become sensitive to guilt and this extremely heightened feeling inside of me. A lot of pain and confusion has come from this because I didn't understand what was happening inside of me... I shall have to work to be able to understand and articulate. In time I will achieve this, but for the moment I am riding my bicycle without a chain.'

About nine months after writing this letter, he wrote another on the occasion of the death of his younger sister, from which the following are extracts:

'This has been a very challenging time and an opportunity for me to practice the issues of bereavement I learned with you last year. I was able to help the rest of my family though the range of emotions associated with grief as I had learnt them. I took an active role in helping to organise the funeral as my family were upset. People often said 'I was coping very well', but they don't understand that emotionally I am at a distance and that it will only be in the future that I may suffer as I finally work the grief out.

'But for the moment I am trying to do the right things. I visited my sister a few times while she was in the mortuary and when I hugged her I got upset because this was the only time I could do this. It upset me that I could hug an inanimate person but not when she was alive. I placed photos and a gold chain in the coffin so I could always remember this in future when my feelings finally understand what has happened. I also made some booklets for the funeral so that she would always be remembered. But for now all I can do is carry on with my life and try to be the best I can.

'Once again, thank you for making me aware about bereavement and helping me to do the right thing while I had the opportunity. Otherwise I would have done nothing and would probably have felt guilty.'

References

At the time of updating this resource anything from, or recommended by, Sheila Hollins or Irene Tuffrey-Wijne would appear to be a good resource.

Attwood, T. (1993). *Why does Chris do that?* London: The National Autistic Society. Available from www.autism.org.uk/pubs.

Attwood, T. (1998). *Asperger's syndrome: a guide for parents and professionals*. London: Jessica Kingsley Publishers. Available from www.autism.org.uk/amazon.

Attwood, T. (1999). Personal correspondence with author.

Attwood, T. (2000). Strategies for improving the social integration of children with Asperger syndrome. *Autism*, 4(1), pp85-100.

Blackman, N. (2003). *Loss and learning disability.* London: Worth Publishing.

Bogdashina, O. (2006). *Theory of mind and the triad of perspectives on autism and Asperger syndrome.* London: Jessica Kingsley Publishers.

Breaking Bad News website: www.breakingbadnews.org.

Brelstaff, K. (1984). Reactions to death: can the mentally handicapped grieve? Some experiences of those who did. *Teaching and training*, 22(1), pp10-16.

Carr, A. T. (1988). 'Dying and bereavement' in Hall, J. (Ed.) *Psychology for nurses and health visitors*, chapter 7. London: Macmillan.

Cathcart, F. (1994). *Understanding death and dying* (three booklets). 1. Your feelings; 2. A guide for family and friends; 3. A guide for carers and other professionals. Kidderminster: British Institute for Learning Disabilities.

Cruse Bereavement Care website: www.cruse.org.uk.

Day, K. (1985). Psychiatric disorder in the middle-aged and elderly mentally handicapped. *British Journal of Psychiatry*, 147, pp660-667.

Department of Health (2005a). *The Mental Capacity Act 2005 – summary*. London: The Stationery Office.

Department of Health (2005b). *The Mental Capacity Act – chapter 9*. London: The Stationery Office.

Dickenson, D. and Johnson, M. (Eds.) (1993). *Death, dying and bereavement*. London: Sage Publications.

Emerson, P. (1977). Covert grief reactions in mentally retarded clients. *Mental Retardation*, 15(6), 46-47.

Gerland, G. (1999). Letter to the Editor: 'Autism and psychodynamic theories'. *Autism*, 3(3), pp309-311.

Giarelli, E. and Gardner, M. (2012). *Nursing of autism spectrum disorder: evidence-based integrated care across the lifespan*. New York: Springer Publishing Company.

Gillberg, C. (1991). Clinical and neurobiological aspects of Asperger syndrome in six family studies. In Frith, U. (Ed.). *Autism and Asperger syndrome*, chapter 4, pp122-146. Cambridge: Cambridge University Press.

Gray, C. (1998). 'Social stories and comic strip conversations with students with Asperger syndrome and high-functioning autism'. In Schopler, E. Mesibov, G. B., Kunce, L. J. (Eds.) *Asperger syndrome or high-functioning autism?* pp167-198. New York: Plenum.

The Gray Center (accessed 28 May 2013): www.thegraycentre.org/social-stories.

Gulbenkoglu, H. (2007). *Supporting people with learning disabilities coping with grief and loss*. Melbourne: Scope (Vic) Ltd.

Handley, E. and Hutchinson, N. (2012). The experience of carers in supporting people ewith intellectual disabilities through the process of bereavement: An interpretative phenomological analysis. *Journal of Applied Research in Intellectual Disabilities*, 26, pp186-194.

Harris, P. (1998). *What to do when someone dies*. London: Which?

Hayworth, M. (1996). Explaining death. In Ward, B. *Good grief*

(2), pp34-36. London: Jessica Kingsley Publishers.

Heslop, P. et al (2013). *Confidential enquiry into the premature deaths of people with learning disabilities (CIPOLD)*. London: Norah Fry Research Centre.

Hollins, S. and Sireling, L. (1994). *When Dad died*. London: St George's Mental Health Library.

Hollins, S. and Sireling, L. (1999). *Understanding grief; working with grief and people who have learning disabilities*. Brighton: Pavilion.

Hollins, S. and Tuffrey-Wijne, I. (2009). *Am I going to die?* London: RSPsych Publications/St George's, University of London.

Johnston, A. *When I die*. Visit www.easyhealth.org.uk (downloaded March 2013).

Jordon, R. and Powell, S. (1995). *Understanding and teaching children with autism*. Chichester: Wiley.

Kane, B. (1997). Children's concepts of death. *Journal of Genetic Psychology*, 134, pp141-153.

Kitching, N. (1987). Helping people with mental handicaps cope with bereavement. *Mental Handicap*, 15, June, pp60-63.

Kübler-Ross, E. (2005). *On grief and grieving: finding the meaning of grief through the five stages of loss*. New York: Simon & Schuster Ltd.

Lansdown, R. (1996). Working with young people facing death. In Ward, B. *Good grief* (2), pp32-33. London: Jessica Kingsley Publishers.

Madders, T. (2010). *You need to know*. London: The National Autistic Society. Available from www.autism.org.uk/reports.

Marie Curie Cancer Care (2012). *Bereavement: helping you to deal with the death of someone close to you*. London: Marie Curie Cancer Care.

McCormick, J. (1998). Growing up - tackling depression. *The autistic spectrum – a handbook*, 1999, pp64-69. London: The National Autistic Society.

McLoughlin, I. J. (1986). Care of the dying: bereavement in the mentally handicapped. *British Journal of Hospital Medicine,* 36(4), pp256-260.

Medley, S. and Saunders, J. (2006). Providing end-of-life care for people with learning disabilities. *Nursing Times*, 102, p21.

Morgan, H. (1996). *Adults with autism: a guide to theory and practice*. Cambridge: Cambridge University Press.

Murdy, J. and O'Leary, L. (1999). Understanding the issues of palliative care for someone with a learning disability. In Blackman, N. (Ed.) *Living with loss, helping people with learning disabilities to cope with bereavement and loss*, pp37-39. Brighton: Pavilion.

National Council for Palliative Care (2009). *Good decision- making: the Mental Capacity Act and end of life care.* Available from www. ncpc.org.uk

Oswin, M. (1991). *Am I allowed to cry? A study of bereavement amongst people who have learning difficulties.* London: Souvenir Press.

Parkes, C. M. (1996). *Bereavement, studies of grief in adult life.* London: Routledge.

Parkes, C. M., Laugani, P., and Young, B. (Eds.) (1997). *Death and bereavement across cultures.* London: Routledge.

Parsons, J. and Sims, P. (2010). *Advocacy for adults with autism spectrum disorders.* London: The National Autistic Society. Available from www.autism.org.uk/pubs.

Peberdy, A. (1993). Spiritual care of dying people. In Dickenson, D. and Johnson, M. (Eds.) *Death, dying and bereavement*, pp219-223. London: Sage Publications.

Pincus, L. (1961). Understanding loss. In Ward, B. (1996). *Good grief (2)*, pp17-19. London: Jessica Kingsley Publishers.

Prior, M. (2000). Editorial. *Autism*, 4(1), pp5-8.

Rawlings, D. (1996, unpublished). *Have I finished being sad?*

Rawlings, D. (1998, unpublished). *An investigation into the effects of bereavement in adults with autism living in residential care services, and an examination of the implications for service providers.*

Read, S. (1998). The palliative care needs of people with learning disabilities. *International Journal of Palliative Nursing*, 4(5), pp246-251.

Read, S. et al (2012). Using action research to design bereavement software: engaging people with intellectual disabilities for effective development. *Journal of Applied Research in Intellectual Disabilities*, 26, pp195-206.

Rutten, A (2007). Counselling. In *Approaches to autism*, p 21. London: The National Autistic Society.

Schuhow, D. and Zurakowski, T. (2013). Evidence based care of the older client with autism. In Giarelli, E. and Gardner, M. (Eds.). *Nursing of autism spectrum disorder*, chapter 14, pp353-385. New York: Springer Publishing Company.

Schaeffer, D. and Lyons, C. (1998). *How do we tell the children?* New York: Newmarket Press.

Sims, P. (2011). *Mental health and autism: a guide for child and adolescent mental health practitioners.* London: The National Autistic Society. Available from www.autism.org.uk/pubs.

Sireling, L. (1989). Life after death (unpublished paper), quoted in Kitching, N. (1987). Helping people with mental handicaps cope with bereavement. *Mental Handicap*, 15, June, pp60-63.

Skylight Trust (2007). *Breaking bad news to children and teens.* Newton: Skylight Trust. Available from www.skylight.org.nz/uploads/files/breaking_bad_news_to_children_and_teens.pdf (downloaded 27 May 2013).

Standard Medical Advisory Committee (SMAC) and Standing Nurse and Midwifery Advisory Committee (1992). *The principles of palliative care. Joint report of SMAC and Standing Nurse and Midwifery Advisory Committee.* London: SMAC.

Staudacher, C. (1988). *Beyond grief, a guide for recovering from the death of a loved one.* London: Souvenir Press.

Stickney, D. (1984). *Waterbugs and dragonflies.* London: Mowbray.

Tantam, D. (2000). Psychological disorder in adolescents and adults with Asperger syndrome. *Autism,* 4(1), pp47-62.

Todd, S. (2012). Being there: the experiences of staff in dealing with matters of dieing and death in services for people with intellectual disabilities. *Journal of Applied Research in Intellectual Disabilities* 2013, 26, pp215-230.

Tuffrey-Wijne, I. (1997). Palliative care and learning disabilities. *Nursing Times*, 93(31), pp50-51.

Tuffrey-Wijne, I. (2013). *How to break bad news to people with intellectual disabilities*. London: Jessica Kingsley Publishers.

Turner, M. (1998). *Talking with children and young people about death and dying, a workbook*. London: Jessica Kingsley Publishers.

Ward, B. et al (1996). *Good grief (2): exploring feelings, loss and death with over elevens and adults*. London: Jessica Kingsley Publishers.

Wertheimer, A. (2001). *A special scar: the experiences of people bereaved by suicide*. London: Routledge.

Wolff, S. (1995). *Loners: the life path of unusual children.* London: Routledge.

Worden, J. W. (1991). *Grief counselling and grief therapy, a handbook for the mental health practitioner.* London: Routledge.

Yanok, J. and Beifus, J. A. (1993). Communicating about loss and mourning: death education for individuals with mental retardation. *Mental Retardation*, 31(3), pp144-147.

Useful contacts

Action for Advocacy (A4A)
PO Box 31856
Lorrimore Square
London SE17 3XR
Tel: 020 7820 7868
Website: www.actionforadvocacy.org.uk
Find advocates in your local area.

British Institute of Learning Disabilities (BILD)
CampionHouse
Green Street
Kidderminster
Worcestershire DY10 1JL
Tel: 01562 723010
Email: enquiries@bild.co.uk
Website: www.bild.org.uk
BILD promotes ways of working with, and for, people with
learning disabilities. It provides training and publishes books and
journals relating to learning disabilities.

The Compassionate Friends
Tel: 0845 123 2304 (Northern Ireland 02087 788016)
Email: info@tcf.org.uk
Website: www.tcf.org.uk
A charitable organisation dedicated to the support and care of
bereaved parents, siblings, and grandparents who have suffered
the death of a child.

Shadow of Suicide Group
Same contact information as The Compassionate Friends
For parents of children who have taken their own lives.

Cruse Bereavement Care
Unit 01
One Victoria Villas
Richmond
Surrey TW9 2GW
Tel: 0844 477 9400
Email info@cruse.org.uk
Website: www.cruse.org.uk
A national organisation offering help to all bereaved people,
including counselling, social meetings and advice on practical
matters. Whenever possible, enquirers are directed to a local
branch – details of which are on Cruse's website.

The National Autistic Society
393 City Road
London EC1V 1NG
Autism Helpline: 0808 800 4104
Email: nas@nas.org.uk
Website: www.autism.org.uk
The UK's leading charity for people with autism, their parents,
carers and family members, and the professionals who work
with them.

The Samaritans
The Upper Mill
Kingston Road
Ewell
Surrey KT17 2AF
Tel: 08457 909090
Email: admin@samaritans.org.uk
Website: www.samaritans.org.uk
A national service for anyone who feels desperate, lonely or suicidal, or who is going through a personal crisis, such as a bereavement.

Humanist and non-religious funerals/cremations

British Humanist Association
39 Morelands Street
London EC1V 8BB
Tel: 020 7324 3060
Email: info@humanism.org.uk
Website: www.humanism.org.uk
Supports those who wish to live humanist lives, including through the provision of humanist ceremonies.

National Secular Society
25 Red Lion Square
London WC1R 4RL
Tel: 020 7404 3126
Email: admin@secularism.org.uk
Website: www.secularism.org.uk

Support for the dying

Help the Hospices
Hospice House
34-44 Britannia Street
London WC1X 9JG
Tel: 020 7520 8200
Email: info@helpthehospces.org.uk
Website: www.helpthehospices.org.uk
Intelligence Hub: www.helpthehospices.org.uk/our-services/intelligence-hub
The Intelligence Hub provides information about hospice and palliative care services across the UK.

Macmillan Cancer Support
89 Albert Embankment
London SE1 7UQ
Tel: 0808 808 0000
Email: information_line@macmillan.org.uk
Website: www.macmillan.org.uk
Macmillan nurses work in hospitals and in the community
throughout the UK.
The service is available to NHS patients via referral by their GP
or district nurse. Some Macmillan nurses specialise in particular
cancers.

Marie Curie Cancer Care
89 Albert Embankment
London SE1 7TP
Tel: 020 7599 7777
Email: info@mariecurie.org.uk
Website: www.mariecurie.org.uk
Marie Curie nurses give practical nursing care to people with
cancer, free of charge. Referral is through a GP or district nurse.
Palliative care is provided in ten Marie Curie centres.

**Palliative Care for People with Learning Disabilities
Network (PCPLD)**
Email: info@pcpid.org
Website: www.pcpid.org
The PCPLD Network brings together service providers, carers,
and people with a learning disability who have palliative care
needs. It offers training and accessible information.